YoU.

BeUtiful

Body

...a guide to eating and loving your body LIGHT

Laura Holland

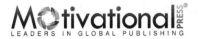
M tivational PRESS®
LEADERS IN GLOBAL PUBLISHING

Published by Motivational Press, Inc.
1777 Aurora Road
Melbourne, Florida, 32935
www.MotivationalPress.com

ISBN: 978-1-62865-506-3

Contents

Part 3 - You and Your Body 90

Part 4 - You and U 111

Part 5 - Weight - The Whole Truth. 120

To BeU is BeUtiful

If there is magic; it's in Being U!

Preface

Relentless dieting, food fearing and body shaming! Uncomfortable, yet all too familiar territory through my teens and early twenties, when even the slightest thought about my body, weight, or food took over my mind. A Starbucks cappuccino and croissant were enough to send me into a state of consuming anxiety for the rest of the day. Obsessing about how many calories I'd just eaten and what I would have to skip eating later to make up for that moment of perceived weakness. Crazy behaviour, especially when you consider that 95% of all weight loss diets fail[1.] Yes, that's right, fail, and that "calories have nothing to do with gaining weight"[2], so counting them to try and lose weight is completely redundant! Also, to be honest, you know something is wrong when a Starbucks triggers a spiraling sense of stress induced bloating and visions of spontaneously expanding two dress sizes!

It is exhausting to constantly criticize your body, not liking this and not liking that, wishing this was smaller, wishing they were bigger! It's a whirlwind of chaos, which leaves you feeling so uncomfortable that you can't even bare to relax in your own skin, let alone your skinny jeans! Throw in a few bad relationships with yourself, your body, and food, and you have a recipe for a total body nightmare, a melt down of all logic and reason, and a blackout to even the tiniest glimmer of your light or natural beauty.

You're right. It is big, and it effects every aspect of your life. A shocking 75% of American women experience unhealthy thoughts, feelings or behaviors related to food or their bodies.[3] That's 75% of women body shaming themselves.

I had a miserable relationship with my body that spilled over into a very challenging relationship with food, and all of this just made for one stressed out, tired, and heavy feeling body, mind, and soul. I had become so entrenched in my tunnel vision of diets and "must-lose-weight" mantra that I couldn't see the wood for the trees. I was so disconnected from my nature, and had no idea how I could begin to change the way I felt about myself or food, let alone get the body I wanted.

It is so sad when you consider the complete dishonoring of ourself inherent in all this stress and negativity. It's a crime we commit daily against ourselves. It is abusive, and there is nothing pretty about it. How can we expect our body to radiate beauty and feel light when it's trapped within such an abusive environment as we adopt a diet mentality that is endemic in today's weight loss culture? Even more importantly, how can we expect it to be healthy and dis-ease free?

The global market for weight loss was worth USD148.1 billion in 2014[4], and it's growing, meanwhile, childhood obesity has tripled since the 1980's[5] whilst anorexia in girls aged 15 - 19 years has increased every decade since the 1930's.[6]

When faced with this reality, can we really afford to ignore the truth of what we are doing to ourselves?

From me to you...

I know what it's like to be so unhappy with the way you think your body looks that you don't know which diet plan to turn to next, having tried them all and still being no closer to the body you desperately want. The irritation inside feels like you should be giving the one minute warning to anyone within a hundred yard radius to avoid the tsunami of frustration that is in danger of being released!

It's tiring and exhausting to live this way, unhappy in your own skin and miserable about your body, it drains your energy and slowly eats away at every last sparkle of life and lightness. Ironically, we may feel full and heavy, but deep down we are starving.

But it doesn't have to be like this. It may be difficult to comprehend, especially if you're in the midst of a constant state of yo-yo dieting, but it is possible to find peace in your skin and feel lighter in your body, and it has nothing to do with dieting as you know it! If you are willing to look in a new direction, through kinder eyes, it will not take as long as you think. By the end of this book you will know how!

I always thought it was interesting that I could experience temporary relief from my diet craziness whilst traveling. I love to travel, food for the soul, literally. It helped me to learn so much more about life, other people, and ultimately myself.

This planet is staggeringly beautiful. If you are yet to discover this for yourself, then get out there and take a good look around.

Mother Nature has to be the ultimate designer of beauty which awes and inspires, with immense diversity, and yet an over-whelming sense of balance prevails.

There is something magical about witnessing the awesome beauty of mountains, oceans, and all the incredible landscapes in-between. Their energy touches you at your core, you feel them and they feel you. This connection is nothing short of transformational. Momentarily, you see and feel something beyond your ordinary perception of life, yourself, and your body.

The Chinese Proverb says "when sleeping women wake, mountains move". I think mountains can help awaken sleeping women, or at least this has been part of my experience. Even the subtlest of sensations as to our true nature is powerful, and we don't have to go all the way to the Himalayas to experience it, we can ask the mountains to come to us!

My growing awareness of the abundant beauty of nature as I travelled the world, slowly opened my eyes to glimpses of the beauty of my own nature and of my body. Being surrounded by nature is powerful. It clears the muddy waters of self criticism and judgement so that you 'see' more clearly.

In a world where beauty is abundant, it would be our greatest misfortune to remain blind to the beauty within us.

My Journey with My Body and Food

Nowadays I love food, good food, but this hasn't always been true. As a Nutritional Therapist, I'm passionate about healthy food and its healing powers, although this hasn't always been the case either. I used to be an Economist, and put my love of numbers to extensive use, micro analyzing every last mouthful of food. Needless to say, this predisposition was not at all helpful and compounded my OCD tendencies when it came to 'managing' my weight. I say I love food, but truthfully I didn't experience the 'love' in this relationship for the longest time. Eating created huge surges of anxiety and discomfort, followed by tremendous guilt after meals, or even just a snack.

Eating was an emotional roller coaster, love hate, literally! Any pleasure I got from eating was quickly eaten up by guilt and fear, followed by feeling so uncomfortable in my clothes. Skinny jeans were the absolute worst, and always forced me into cosy PJ's at every opportunity, regardless of the time of day, in an attempt to cover the crime that I had just committed. Life is just not fun when you live with this kind of sentence around food.

With three emotional roller coasters a day, or less on serious 'diet days', you can see that obsessing about food, my body, and weight took up huge portions of my day. I spent so much time feeling bad about myself, I literally had no time to think about anything good! I wreaked havoc in my physical body and my wellbeing suffered.

Thankfully, I did wake-up from all of this craziness. I reached my limit of discomfort, coupled with feeling heavy, no matter what I ate, always miserable around food, regardless of my dress size, so enough was enough! Something inside of me knew this wasn't right, this was not the way I was supposed to be living or eating.

I had exhausted all conceivable dieting scenarios and came to a point where there were two clear and distinct choices before of me. First, I could continue down this same path, hating my body, being terrified of food, becoming more miserable and depressed about my body and inevitably reaching the scary realms of extreme diet yo-yoing, and still being no closer to the body I wanted. Or, I could surrender, release the struggle, lay down my weapons of self-destruction and end this inner 'war on terror' that had waged inside me for far too long. It was clear that those were my only options, two paths, one heading further into the nightmare and the other heading in the opposite direction, the known versus the unknown, I chose the latter.

Every cell in my body was telling me that what I had been doing up to this point was wrong, and it was within a rare moment of stillness that I finally heard my body scream to me "enough is enough." I had felt powerless for, what felt like, forever, but I did have the power to make a different choice and, in that moment, for the first time, I realized it.

Do you want to wake up from your body nightmare?

We have come too far in our understanding, with increasing awareness of the laws of the universe and how our body is manifest, to keep stuck on the idea of "no-pain no-gain" exercise regimes and "no-carb low-calorie" diet plans. Something is missing, ironically, a seriously large piece of the pie hasn't been eaten, and it isn't the kale!

How many times have you asked yourself 'how do I lose this weight?' And I bet you've said to yourself 'what's wrong with my body?' These two questions are dangerous, don't ever ask them again! They're part of the problem because they are completely devoid of self-love and lack even the slightest comprehension of the true process of your body, whilst being stacked with all the weight of previous diets that have left you feeling frustrated and heavy. Instead, ask 'how can

I begin to feel lighter?' Then ask 'what's my body trying to tell me?' A subtle difference but one that sets you on a completely different trajectory.

Through my journey, and with all the women I've worked with, self-love is nearly always missing, or seriously deficient, and it just so happens to be the single most important ingredient for a light feeling body. Love is the most powerful nutrient that we can feed ourselves, and, is essential if we are to find the balance needed for a healthy, beautiful body.

If there was just one message that I want you to get from reading this book, and coming on this journey with me, it would be this - there is nothing wrong with you or your body, but there is something wrong with your thinking!

You need to start using your own guidance rather than just following what everyone else is doing, or eating whatever the latest diet plan says you need to eat. By connecting and listening to the wisdom of your own body, then taking inspired action, you find your balance and this is the most powerful position from which to effortlessly create your most beautiful body, naturally.

It is a revelation for me to be able to just Be, to eat and not be filled with anxiety, guilt and heaviness. To just Be me, free from my mentally created stress and prison of distorted reality is nothing short of revolutionary, and now I am going to help you to experience this freedom and feel light, in your body, mind and soul.

Your Journey

"What you seek is seeking you."
Rumi

This isn't a diet, or an eating plan telling you what to eat, when and how much. I am not trying to get you to a certain size or weight, I don't care what your dress size is or what the scales say. What I do care about is how you feel, and I want you to feel light, because how you feel is what you live.

This is a different kind of nutrition, inspired by your body wisdom, with an intuitive approach to eating, a deeper level of understanding of food, its energy, and its alchemical potential, whilst understanding the power of your mind and emotions in creating your physical body.

To eat is a pleasure, but to eat well is an art! The artistry here is in the creation of balance within your body, mind and soul as you eat. It is this balance, or alignment, with your Self, that facilitates the type of lightness you are really seeking. But to create this balance, you have to know where you are, physically, emotionally and energetically. So your journey is within - within your body, within your mind, within your emotions, within the very fabric of your Being, nurturing an awareness of yourself that brings intention and meaning to each mouthful of food.

I will guide you through an 8 week BeUtiful body holistic process, tuning into how your body functions so you can finally work with your body, rather than against it, creating the state of health and body that you desire.

In preparation for these 8 weeks we will address emotional comfort eating, understand how to eat to feel calmer, reduce stress, enhance digestion, balance your hormones and nurture your adrenal and thyroid function, and most importantly, learn how to love food, your body and yourself. We will also embrace metaphysical principles that have been completely left out of all mainstream diets, and learn how to put the theory into practice.

Whilst this is a journey of feeling light and creating your most BeUtiful Body, at the heart of everything you're about to read, is to help you to connect more fully with your Self. This is where your creative power is, with the potential for complete, inner and outer, transformation, because if there is magic, and I believe there is, it is in Being U!

Each chapter is an opportunity for you to connect more deeply with your body. I will guide you through self-care practices, rituals, nutritional wisdom, mantras and meditations. By the time you have finished this book and experienced the 8 week BeUtiful body process, you will be love-filled, feeling lighter and awake to the beauty that you are.

My intention is to help you to hear your body wisdom and then guide you in making intuitive choices about food, exercise and how to work with your body, in an intelligent and inspired way. Gently guiding you back into a state of balance, on all levels. Feeling light and beautiful are the natural, logical, consequences of a balanced state. Why? Because, in a balanced state you align with your true nature and the nature of the cosmos - light energy. In your balanced, aligned state, this is what you allow to flow through you, and it clears all dis-ease and heaviness in its path.

"The cosmos is within us, we are made of star stuff."

Carl Sagan

This book will change you in more ways than you're expecting, and if you are reading this then I have no doubt that deep down you have been searching for more. We need to break-free from the limiting beliefs about food and dieting that are keeping us trapped in body's that we can't make peace with, because this is what's stopping us from feeling light and beautiful.

We are in need of a diet evolution to inspire a beauty revolution. So, if we can wake-up and open our minds to ultimate reality - how we are the creators of our life, how we determine our health and how we shape our body, every single inch of it, we can stop being distracted by a restrictive diet culture that's wreaking havoc with our wellbeing and reclaim our body sovereignty. The time for this is Now, so let's get started.

Part 1 - Let There Be Light

Diets: Why Not?

The short answer, is because 95% of people that go on a diet fail to lose weight!'

We have to admit, the majority of us get no closer to the body we want after a diet. We also gain an acute awareness of what we don't like about our body. The 'diet drama' then turns up a few notches as our attention gets stuck on all the parts of our body we're not feeling the love for, compounded by, what feels like, despite our best efforts 'those bits' not budging an inch!

For some of us, 'dieting' can then take on a more sinister form as our body image plummets! According to a study published by Philadelphia Eating Disorder Examiner, 35% of "occasional dieters" progress into pathological dieting, or disordered eating, and as many as 25% into full blown eating disorders.

The fact that there are so many diets is a clue that they don't work too well. If they did, then I'm guessing there would not be so many of them! Surely one would be enough?

Diets breed fear around food and an un-natural approach to eating, which has taken us further away from our most natural state of feeling healthy and light. Addressing the food you eat certainly has a place when it comes to weight and health, and we will be dealing with this later, but it should never be within the context of a diet mentality. Diet mentality usually has no appreciation of how your body functions and is solely concerned with getting you thinner. However, it completely fails to realize that for your body to get rid of excess weight that it's holding on to, your body has to be functioning optimally, and, when it does, weight will naturally take care of itself.

Diets are also based on a restriction mindset and let's be honest, restriction does not feel good. As humans we are instinctively drawn to freedom and expansion. So, when we approach our eating from this restrictive mindset, we are always careful to stay 'in control' and not go 'off plan', which creates a constant battle within. Food literally becomes the enemy.

What we eat is one of the few things that we feel is totally within our control, but when we diet we give this sense of control away, leaving us feeling more like a victim to food, as our natural eating habits become distorted.

Before you know it, you're weighing your cereals, counting calories, saving points so you can 'cheat' at the weekend, and stockpiling anything with 'low fat' on the label, regardless of whether you like it or not. You make choices on what to eat based upon its calorie content, irrespective of whether it's healthy for your body, or even if it tastes good.

There are four major problems with this diet mentality:

1. Dieting is a completely unnatural way of thinking about food and making choices about what to eat, which usually results in your body feeling unnourished, unsupported and unloved. It lets you know all of this by feeling tired, bloated, agitated and heavy. Good does not come from doing something that feels bad. Your body wants to eat what it needs in order to function optimally and thrive, nothing more and nothing less. This is what should be guiding what you eat, not a diet plan, because you are unique and your needs are different to everybody else's.

2. You give power away to food when you wrongly believe that your weight is solely a product of the food you eat. A self-fulfilling prophecy, that creates fear and negativity around eating, as you forget your inner knowing of the healing potential of food and how to eat and receive essential nourishment. When you don't give your body what it needs, it will hold on to everything else!

3. Restriction and a dieting mindset makes your body hypersensitive to food and your weight fluctuates all over the place, making it more difficult to feel 'in control' of. One weekend of eating 'off plan' is enough to get you straight back to square one when you step on those scales Monday morning.

4. With all of this negative focus on food, trying to diet becomes a battle of willpower and sheer determination to avoid 'bad' foods. Whilst you may want to remain steadfast in the 'just say no' policy for particular foods, their temptation grows exponentially to match your willpower, and it is only a matter of time, usually when you've had a stressful day, that your willpower fails you, and the rest of the day is spent feeling guilty, bloated and heavy, perpetuating a negative cycle of yo-yo dieting and feeling bad about yourself.

I have lost count of the number of times my clients have said that eating 'healthy' is hard work. These people are not lying, they're telling the truth from their perspective. But we can become so obsessed with diets and weight, that avoiding 'problem foods' so desperately, can actually make them impossible to avoid. What we resist persists. Pushing against something that you don't want doesn't get rid of it, it usually brings it closer.

Also, each of us are unique. What creates balance and lightness in you may do the complete opposite in me. We have to stop following diets blindly under this 'one-size-fits-all' mentality. To find your balance your body has to be at the heart of every single decision you make. Otherwise, how do you know if something, like food for example, is helping or hurting your body? A book can't tell you that, only you can. That's the problem with diets and living so fast that your head is miles ahead of your body.

These diets don't know your body, and neither do you because you're completely unaware of what your body is trying to tell you. You have to become aware of what creates balance, and what doesn't, in each moment, for your body. A salad is not always the answer, believe me, I have seen more clients with digestive issues exasperated by obsessive salad eating than you can imagine.

Get Off The Scales

Daily weigh-ins and diets go hand-in-hand, but they are completely counterproductive, only serving to keep you trapped within diet mentality. The numbers don't mean anything anyway; your happiness with your body shouldn't be based on something external like what the scales said this morning.

In my late teens and early twenties I had to visit the doctor every six months to have my blood pressure and weight checked because I was taking the contraceptive pill. On one of those occasions I went in there feeling absolutely fine and comfortable in my body and we went through the usual process. This time, after she'd weighed me she said, rather abruptly, that I was five pounds heavier than I was six months ago and I should "definitely try to lose it before it got too much for me to lose!" I walked out of there feeling totally depressed and fat! For perspective, I was no bigger than a UK size twelve at the time. This triggered months of yo-yo dieting and feeling miserable about my body and food, until I finally managed to regain my balance again.

Setting aside the fact that my 'heavier' weight was probably nothing to do with how much I was eating and more likely due to hormonal imbalance and side-effects from taking the pill, the reality is, I probably would have regained my balance a lot quicker, and naturally, if I hadn't reacted to the weigh-in quite so sensitively and instantly judged my body. So, until you have de-sensitized yourself to those numbers on the scales, stay away! Because getting on there and feeling bad about it is not going to get you lighter anytime soon.

Also, just to add, who still thinks it's a good idea to treat a hormone imbalance by adding synthetic hormones into your body? It may be good for pharmaceutical businesses, but it certainly is not a good idea for female health.

Weight naturally fluctuates, especially for women, depending on hormonal cycles, the seasonal cycles of the year and what's going on in your life right now, for example, how much sleep you are getting and your stress levels. The more you try to control the number, the more elusive it becomes. Just give your mind, and body, a rest from the scales for a while. Practice tuning in to how your body feels, how you feel in your clothes, how comfortable you feel in your skin and take your lead from this, your body wisdom.

For the rest of our time working together through this book please avoid weighing yourself to judge your progress. Instead focus on how your body is feeling and use this as your guide as you begin to tune into your body with greater understanding and more love.

Stop Counting Calories

After years of being told that we need to get counting calories if we want to lose weight, I understand what a shock to the system it is to stop the food arithmetic.

I have had this discussion so many times, but believe me, calories are not the bottom-line. My background is economics and I love numbers. I would be super happy if weight was just a simple matter of eating a set amount of calories. The fact is, it isn't. Not all calories are equal, and each body is different with much more going on than this simplistic equation of calories in and calories out.

One of my favorite health and wellness professionals, Dr Mark Hyman, tells us that "the vast majority of conventional nutritionists and doctors have it mostly wrong when it comes to weight loss", and the "biggest lie" promoted through mainstream media and the diet industry is that "all calories are created equal". He explains that "some calories are addictive, others healing, some fattening, some metabolism boosting. That's because food doesn't just contain calories, it contains information"! He then goes on to use the example of a study of 154 countries that looked at the correlation of adding 150 calories per day to the diet and it barely raised the risk of diabetes, but, if those 150 calories came from soda the risk of diabetes went up by 700%.

Also, calorie counting is such an unnatural way of eating, our ancestors didn't count calories, they didn't need to, their food was all natural rather than manufactured products.

When you try to diet by continuously cutting calories as part of your everyday eating, you may lose weight initially but your body will get used to operating at this lower caloric intake level and eventually you have to undercut your calories even more to lose weight.

This can only go one way, inevitably ending with you hardly eating anything, feeling weak, irritable and starving. To make things worse, your metabolism has also slowed down and your body has switched into starvation mode, this means that everything you eat is now being stored. You could even find yourself gaining a little weight and bloating, especially around your middle as your body becomes stressed and tries to protect itself. You won't be able to continue at this low calorie diet without seriously harming your digestion and creating significant stress. Both of these situations will make you very sensitive to gaining weight quickly, whilst pushing you further away from a light, comfortable feeling stomach. You're also more likely to be under nourished, since counting calories usually means a lack of nutrients.

A client once came to me because she was desperate to lose weight for her wedding. In the first session I always ask my clients to explain to me what they're eating so I can understand where we are and how their bodies are reacting so to begin designing a way forward relative to their unique body and preferences. Tentatively she began to talk me through what she eats in a day, it took her all of a few seconds, she was surviving on less than 600 calories a day, whilst working full time and going to the gym, with a personal trainer (and we know how hardcore they can be so she wasn't slacking there!) four times a week. She was utterly miserable and couldn't shift the weight that she wanted and said "how can I be this size eating this little?"

There are some people that think that all over-weight people don't work-out and over-eat, they don't, and this is not true. This woman was not lying, she was working her ass off, figuratively not literally, and her body was staying stubbornly at the same weight. She felt her body was against her, she was incredibly frustrated and feeling so down about herself. The wedding was four months away and she was panic stricken with the thought that this is how her body was going to look. Unfortunately the more this had continued the more dislike she had for herself, which only made her body more stressed, more uncomfortable, heavier and bloated.

It is irrelevant what size she was and wanted to be, what was important is how she felt. She felt heavy, uncomfortable and out of control with her body. In her attempt to feel lighter, the dieting and calorie restricting caused more harm, physically and emotionally, intensifying these negative feelings about her body even more. Now her body was stressed and starving, and there is no way that beauty and lightness are going to come from this state.

It was quite a journey that we had together, emotionally undoing the harm she had unleashed on herself in her desperate attempts to feel beautiful for her wedding day. She was incredibly anxious to follow what I wanted her to do, but I finally convinced her to eat a little more, train a little less, eat specific foods that would ease the stress in her body and support her adrenal glands. I taught her to listen to her body, to eat intuitively, to help heal her digestion with specific rituals and herbs. I even got her doing some of my favorite breathing techniques and energy medicine to help improve her digestion, whilst calming her body down so it felt safe enough to let go of what it was holding onto so tightly.

There was slow progress, but it was sure and steady. Most of all however, through our time together, she calmed down, connected to her body, appreciated it more, and began to cultivate a greater sense of love for herself. Her body responded and she looked radiant by the time the wedding day arrived. It is incredible what the right combination of food and self-love can do!

Ironically, the more we count calories, the more we create fear around food and our body. The discomfort we feel is our body trying to let us know how unhappy it feels and how out of balance it has become.

I noticed early in my work with clients that those who were most worried about eating and restricted food usually struggled with weight, whilst those who were more relaxed around food and ate what they wanted seemed to be more comfortable and felt lighter. I know this sounds counterintuitive, but it is true! Counting calories and practicing restrictive eating makes your body hypersensitive to weight gain, further compounding your need to control food. But it's not calories you need to be counting, it's the nutrients.

Nutrients are infinitely more important than calories, you have to eat food to provide your body with these essential 'tools' for your health, wellbeing and to feel light. Using the calorie counter, you'd eat a diet-biscuit rather than a handful of nuts. I promise you right now, nuts, or avocado's for that matter, are not the reason for anyone's excess weight or the increasing obesity rates.

When you learn how to relax around food, eat comfortably, choose foods that feel good to eat, and give your body exactly what it needs to move towards balance, your body will very happily let go of the stuff it no longer needs, it would be inefficient if it didn't, and nature is not inefficient.

However, it is important to recognize that each body is different and the same diet can't, and won't, work for all of us. What creates balance and lightness in your body may be very different from mine. Following a diet totally ignores these differences in all of us, so it is no surprise that diets don't work for all of us in the same way, and this is why it is so important to listen to how your body feels and what it wants to eat.

Eating what you feel your body needs may be scary at first, but real food does not make you fat. That's right, real, natural food does not make you fat.

Most of all, restricting calories doesn't work because you are starving your body of love as you spend your days trying your best to ignore your hunger, basically ignoring yourself, this is self-abandonment. Your body feels unloved, unsupported, and enters into a state of stress. This is definitely not a recipe for love and light, in your mind or in your dress size, and counting calories or points keeps you locked into thinking about quantity when your only concern should be the quality of your food.

The next time you are reading food labels, take a look at the ingredients list and make your decision based on that, not the calorie content. If you are counting calories then you are eating the wrong foods.

I once lost a lot of weight quickly but I was surviving on a diet exclusively of vegetables and fruit. Ironically, I still wasn't happy with my body even though I had lost so much weight. How much more miserable can you get? To add insult to injury I had a bloated tummy most of the time despite being pretty skinny at this point. In retrospect, this was my body screaming to stop. Luckily I was at least eating 'healthy foods' but I'd created a whole lot of stress, tension, anxiety and deprivation in my body. This resulted in adrenal fatigue, thyroid issues and hormonal imbalance. I was totally out of balance and felt extremely disconnected, which only fueled an increasingly negative body image. My body wasn't the problem though, no more than food, I was!

Focus On Light

Throughout this book I will constantly encourage you to focus on feeling light, rather than getting thin or losing weight. Why? Because getting thin and losing weight suggests that 'weight' is the problem - it isn't. Weight is merely a symptom of imbalance, and if the imbalance is ignored, as it most often is in the pursuit of getting thin and losing weight, then you are completely powerless to make any sustainable progress with your weight.

To make matters worse, if your focus is on losing weight, then you're going to be on the scales every morning, measuring your 'success' by a number and paying attention to this, rather than tuning into how your body actually feels.

In reality, weight is a very poor indicator of how healthy you are, how balanced you are and how you feel in your body. Also, for many people the words 'weight loss' are loaded with all the struggle of previous diet attempts. When weight loss is the goal, all of your decisions about food and exercise are focused on this, regardless of how good they feel and how healthy they are for you, with absolutely no appreciation for how your body actually functions.

As for getting thin, well 'thin' and 'light' are two completely different things, you can be 'thin' but feel anything but 'light', and continue destructive dieting in an attempt to get to your idea of what 'thin' is, whilst completely ignoring the health and wellbeing of your own body. With body dysmorphia so prevalent these days, your own judgement of how 'thin' your body looks is often completely skewed, therefore, focusing on 'getting thin' traps you into this external assessment of your body.

Ultimately, the problem with weight loss and getting thin, is that they both lock you into a purely physically focused approach to your body, which in a rather large dose of irony, completely disconnects you from your body and disempowers you in the process.

In contrast, focusing on feeling light turns all of your attention inward, tuning into to how your body feels, and then from this place of conscious awareness being able to make the best, most intelligent choices, relative to food and exercise, that will serve your highest good. You will also be able to address the root causes of heaviness, rather than merely treating weight as the problem.

Also, light energy is essentially what we are made of in terms of physics, so focusing on what we actually are is a much better use of all of our time rather than abstract terms like 'getting thin' and 'weight loss'.

In addition, if you 'feel it' you will 'be it', focusing on feeling light, as opposed to feeling heavy, is the most effective way of helping your body to feel lighter, whatever that may look like for your unique body. Yes, it is more subtle than weight loss and getting thin, but focusing on feeling light is a way of working with your body without suffering the negative consequences of diet mentality.

Dieting and the relentless quest for a mentally constructed idea of the perfect body has been one of the most significant sources of disempowerment for women in modern times, encouraging more and more women, and girls, to negatively judge their body and have dangerously poor body images.

This has lead to disturbing statistics of eating disorders, a massive lack of self-confidence, low self-worth and depression in increasing percentages of the female population. We have to start approaching weight from a completely different perspective to heal the damage done, whilst simultaneously finding ways to reconnect with our natural beauty and All that we are.

It is not an exaggeration to say that the rise of the divine feminine depends upon women embracing their body, loving their body, seeing the beauty within their body and seeing the beauty within each other. There is no more time to 'play small', and this is exactly what diets, weight loss and getting thin induces. Enough! This is why we focus on feeling light.

Stop chasing getting thin and start seeking your light.

What is a BeUtiful Body?

"A cultural fixation on female thinness is not an obsession about female beauty, but an obsession about female obedience. Dieting is the most potent political sedative in women's history; a quietly mad population is a tractable one."

Naomi Wolf

In our lifetime the idea of beauty has become synonyms with thinness. Increasingly manufactured, packaged, labelled and sold, beauty has become a commodity bound by ever decreasing sizes, dimensions and conditions, and the 'cost' of beauty has never been as high as it is today.

As the abundant, unconditional nature of beauty has been slowly eroded, so has the appreciation of the divine feminine, shadowed by the emergence of patriarchal governance of religion and economy. This is completely out of balance, and rooted in fear and ownership rather than equality.

Amidst such inequality and lack of appreciation for each other, fear reigns, and paves the way for judgement and criticism. Today we compare and judge ourselves, trying to imitate a socially constructed idea of the 'perfect body' which doesn't even exist. It is no wonder that we never seem to 'get it', no matter how much we diet, how hard we exercise, or how many lotions and potions we smother ourselves in.

We have this mentally constructed idea in our heads of how we think we should look, fixated on being 'thin' rather than feeling 'light', and we wrestle our body into that 'one-size-fits-all' definition of beauty. But it's just so limiting, it cannot possibly accommodate the sheer diversity and uniqueness that each of us is blessed with. We get trapped in this external search for a beautiful body, and it feels impossible. This is what happens when something as natural as beauty gets controlled, manipulated and packaged into diets, turning it into a wholly un-natural version of what it truly is. Now this 'commodity' has a price, whilst real beauty is priceless.

The artists among us haven't, but the masses, in a super-sized dose of irony, have forgotten that the most beautiful, captivating and even mesmerizing aspect of beauty is that it has no limits or constraints. Beauty is limitless and that is its beauty!

Like love, you are looking for beauty in all the wrong places. This is true no matter how cliché it may sound. Stop your external search, quit the dieting, turn around, and look within yourself. Your beauty starts here and unless you uncover this beautiful seed and nurture it with your own awareness, self-love and care, it will never see the light of day, at least not through your eyes, the only eyes that really matter anyway.

Now more than ever, we all need to empower ourselves by reconnecting to the nature of who-we-really-are and start treating ourselves in a way that is befitting of our divine feminine, naturally beautiful. This is our power, to know who-we-are and connect with the light that we are. Take the word 'thin' out of your vocabulary and replace it with 'light', and seek this.

There is a certain air of confidence that glows from a woman who is connected to her divine feminine energy that is powerful. This woman has tapped into her own 'well of beauty' and allowed it to blossom into her body. I assure you, this woman doesn't stress herself over the latest diet craze and she isn't fixated on thinness or the hottest style that everyone must fit into! She is 'in' her body and loves it, and so, her body is BeUtiful.

A BeUtiful body is your body, your own unique expression of beauty. You will find this body when you go within, to the source of your Being, your light. Once you connect more deeply with yourself and find your balance, you can bring this light to the surface, unhindered by negative thoughts, judgements or harmful foods causing stagnation. Healing all of these 'toxins' along the way, so that by the time you get back to the surface your light is still shining and you're not just feeling it, you are it!

So Who Are U?

I'm sure you've already noticed that I'm blending mainstream nutrition and biology with metaphysical principles. You may be asking yourself what's this got to do with my weight? But I assure you it has everything to do with your weight, and everything else in your life. When you leave these principles out of the equation you disempower yourself from being able to consciously take full creative control of your life - your health becomes a matter of fate, or genetics, rather than you being the creator of the health and weight you experience.

At the root of these metaphysical principles is a broader understanding of who 'you' are, so we need to spend a little time unravelling these layers of 'you', because you are not just the sum of your personality, personal preferences and relationship status.

Not to say all of those things about 'you' aren't important, they are, and living in a way that honors them leads to a happy, healthy, emotionally balanced, feel good life experience. However, if you are growing and evolving, some of these are transient and changeable. So who are 'you' beyond these impermanent characteristics? What is the constant? The constant is source energy, consciousness, vibrational energy, and I refer to this as U, meaning 'you' in the ultimate sense.

So on one level, being you is having an appreciation for your unique personality, preferences, biology, body type and ethnicity, and honoring all of this through your choices. For example, living your truth, being authentic, being honest about how you feel and listening to your body wisdom to understand what your body would like to eat for a greater sense of balance. But that's not all. To be U is also to understand, and know, that essentially you're vibrational energy, just like everything else in this universe. Therefore, to be yourself doesn't just mean living in a way that is aligned with your personal preferences and beliefs, it also means living in a way that is aligned with your ultimate Self - source energy, vital life force - love.

This is the greatest realization we can have. Not only does it have the capacity to shift the way we live, for our individual, collective and environmental wellbeing, understanding that ultimately we are all intrinsically connected, it is also our route to a complete healing of body, mind and soul in the realization that 'we are' already and that everything we want is truly within. In this sense there is nothing to get, and we definitely don't need to 'get thin', we just have to align ourselves with our ultimate Self to allow our natural light and beauty to manifest into our physical body. This is what makes your most BeUtiful body, being U.

It all begins with U...

There is no other place to begin because U are the source, literally, and creating balance physically, mentally and emotionally is how you connect, or align yourself with your source energy. Therefore, all of our work with food, nutrition, exercise and lifestyle that we are going to go through together in this book, is all in the context of helping you to live in a more balanced state.

However, to live a balanced state we have to embrace all pieces of ourselves, which means seeing beyond just the body we don't like and embracing our beliefs, thoughts, emotions, experiences and dreams. All of these pieces are part of ourselves too and all have creative power in the health of our body. But how often do we acknowledge them, let alone embrace them, and we wonder why we can't get rid of a bloated stomach? Yes, the gluten probably isn't helping but, I guarantee you that's only a part of your story.

> *"We are not human beings having a spiritual experience.*
> *We are spiritual beings having a human experience."*
>
> *Pierre Teilhard de Chardin*

It is time that we integrated this wisdom and metaphysical principles into how we work with our physical body, especially when it comes to matters of weight and diets, because we are doing ourselves so much harm by ignoring them.

Now take a deep breath. Pause just for a little while. Have you digested this information? We hardly ever give ourselves the time to take a moment and check in with how something has made us feel.

Now is a good time to begin a BeUtiful Body Journal. Find a notebook that makes you happy when you look at it and label it My BeUtiful Body. On the first page begin to write down whatever comes to mind as you ask yourself this important question:

» *How does it feel to be in your body right now?*

Have you ever even asked yourself how your body feels? Not what you're thinking or projecting on to it, but actually how your body feels? There is no right or wrong answer that you could give to this question, but being consciously aware of your body and your journey through this book is the necessary ingredient for your own inner alchemy to work its magic. If you would have asked me this question a few years ago, my answer would have been littered with critical thoughts and negativity.

If negative thoughts are going through your head right now, don't worry, relax, breathe a little deeper, and just commit to keeping an open mind as we move through this book together. Don't fight those thoughts, and don't get attached to them. Just be conscious of where you are right now and be willing to feel it all, without judgement.

This book is an invitation for you to become more conscious of what you are feeding your body, not just food, but your thoughts. Knowledge is power. When you understand what is happening and how your body is being created, you have an opportunity to make new choices.

I know this may seem challenging. After all, many of us, myself included, have spent the majority of our life since teenage years body shaming and criticizing every last inch of our waistline. I for one, have exhausted all possible criticisms you could possibly conjure up for your thighs. But just because this is what we have been doing, does not mean that we must continue.

This negative way of thinking has induced treatment of our body that has created unprecedented levels of poor body image and disordered eating. If we want to create something different then it isn't our body that needs to change, it's our mind and the way we think.

"We cannot solve our problems with the same thinking we used when we created them."

Albert Einstein

Self-deprecation all too easily becomes a habit, socially acceptable, even encouraged, and it's catching! Years ago women fought for our voices to be heard, how terrible would it be if today those voices were being used to criticize our body and other women's?

Research shows that poor body image is related to the onset of depression, eating disorders, poor development and interpersonal skills, negative self-esteem, unhealthy exercise regimes, substance abuse and unhealthy dieting[8]. So, if we don't like our body, then there is a high probability that other areas of our life are going to be negatively impacted. For example, low self-esteem and a lack of confidence taint our efforts to chase our dreams, so fulfilling our life potential becomes much harder when we are experiencing life in a body we feel miserable about - all that incredible potential has a higher probability of remaining trapped inside.

Conversely, when you feel good, when you love and appreciate your body, you feel confident and like everything is possible. You look on the positive side of life with a "can do" attitude. You put your dreams into action because you believe in your ability. You're happy and you feel good, this attracts more happiness and good feelings to you. This is a powerful position to be in because it is easy, natural even, to unlock your amazing potential and live your heart's desire and soul purpose.

If you want to create your most BeUtiful body you need to get into this latter state, and you do so by finding your balance and aligning with U, with love and appreciation for All that you are.

The Holy Trinity of a BeUtiful Body

Just by delving beneath the surface of diets and body image, we've begun to see that there is more going on than meets the eye, and certainly more than just counting calories, when it comes to feeling light and beautiful.

Let's break this down now so we can understand and formulate this BeUtiful process relative to your body. There are three relationships that are pivotal to your wellbeing and have the power to effect everything in your life experience, including your dress size. They do this whether you are conscious of it or not. If these three relationships are not love-filled, then a beautiful, light, healthy body is practically impossible, regardless of how many veggie juices you're getting through in a week.

Your relationship with food, your body and U. Lets look at each one now -

Your Relationship with Food

In just about every culture and tradition that I have seen or read about, food is central to special times when people come together, and especially during times of celebration.

Trying to separate food from pleasure as many of today's typical diets urge us to do, is not only boring, but completely against what is at the root of our natural relationship with food. Also, we rely upon food for our survival, without it we could not live. So it is absolutely logical and natural that we are going to have a 'relationship' with food.

For centuries, when there has been something to celebrate, food has been used to bring people together, to share in the fruits of Mother Earth and to taste this delicious abundance for which we are thankful. Food is to be enjoyed, we are meant to receive pleasure from food and eating is meant to be pleasure-filled.

We are not robots, it is inevitable that we are going to have an emotional response to what we eat, and denying this is unnatural. Food is a source of pleasure, it is a source of nourishment for our survival, and, with the right choices, it's also healing. However, food is not our only source of pleasure, and this is important to appreciate.

So, we really do need to start loving what we are eating and eating what we are loving, especially if we are what we eat. If we eat and then feel guilty or eat foods that we don't like, how can we expect a positive outcome?

The basic premise of eating is to receive nourishment on all levels, unfortunately modern diet culture has cut us off from this and we are now living the consequences of this disconnection manifesting in ever increasing rates of obesity and diseases.

Healing your relationship with food will allow you to receive the love and nourishment you need to create the necessary environment for your health and BeUtiful body.

Do you feel hungry regardless of what you have eaten? It's not surprising if you have a relationship with food that cuts you off from receiving the nourishment and positive energy that is there for you.

When dieting, you usually feel guilty, anxious and irritated around food. You have more 'fat' thoughts on a diet day than at any other time as you scrupulously dissect the calorific content of every mouthful of food. This kind of relationship is not conducive to happy eating nor a happy body, and an unhappy body can never ever be filled with lightness and peace.

Your Relationship with your Body

How you feel about your body matters, it greatly influences your life experience so caring about how your body feels is not superficial. You can't live in a body that you don't like, with constant negative dialogue, and have a healthy, happy body. Just like you can't be obsessing over your body feeling heavy, and feel light at the same time.

So many times we swing from completely obsessing about how we look, to complete abandonment of any form of self-care and nourishment. But there are few things more important than how we feel about our body, our temple. Notice I refer to how we 'feel' about our body, rather than how we think we 'look'.

How we feel in our body is of vital importance, not because of it's physical appearance, but because of what our body represents. "The oldest, the most profound, the most universal of all symbols is the human body." "The Mysteries of every nation taught that the laws, elements, and powers of the universe were epitomized in the human constitution; that everything which existed outside of man had its analogue within man."[9]

Your body, therefore, is a microcosm of the macrocosm. Basically, the universe! So your relationship with your body is reflective of your relationship with life, and the more love-filled it is, the happier your experience will be. In light of this, it would be an excellent idea to replace all your weight and dress size goals with just one goal - to feel good in your body, because when you think about it, this is at the heart of what you are wanting to achieve. Up until this moment you have just been believing that the only route to feeling good in your body is to 'get thin', it isn't, it's to love your body and feel light.

Coupled with your relationship with food, your relationship with your body influences the choices you make relative to thoughts, food, exercise and lifestyle, all of which have a direct effect on the state of your health, wellbeing and how light you feel.

A client was talking to me about how she decides what to eat and drink. She said that it always seemed easier to choose something that wasn't great for her, like take-outs and fast food. As she was talking I looked at the table where her soda sat, she followed my gaze and said instantly, "I could have just as easily ordered water or juice than a soda couldn't I?" She looked at me confused and obviously feeling down about herself and asked, "why didn't I?" I replied "because everything you choose to eat or drink is just a reflection of how you are feeling about you and your body. That's it. Nothing more and nothing less."

Her visual discomfort began to fade, as for the first time, she could make total sense of her choice, and all her past choices, that she had beaten herself up over and felt completely powerless about. When faced with this simple fact, and in her new found awareness and understanding of her behavior around food, she felt empowered to begin to make small changes. You see, your relationship with your body is completely intertwined with your relationship with food, and vice versa, because how you feel about your body influences whether you choose foods and drinks that heal or harm according to your own beliefs about what is 'healthy' or not. Understanding this creates a window of opportunity to begin making different choices.

What you choose to eat and how, is a mirror to how you feel about your body, and this is why it is important to make sure your relationship with your body is focused on love.

Your Relationship with U

Your relationship with U is the most sacred relationship of all. It is the starting point because U are the source, and your relationship with U is really your relationship with everything else.

In many ways it is irrelevant what you eat, and what you think about your body, if you don't 'like' U. I mean it is practically impossible to think loving thoughts about your body and eat in a way that nourishes and nurtures you if you don't love and approve of yourself. If you don't accept U, love U, and honor U, there is always something missing that prevents you coming from a place of love for your body.

When you don't like yourself, you feel more disconnected and everything that you do feels like hard work and effort. It's when no matter how little you eat or how much you run yourself ragged on the treadmill, your body stays stubbornly at the same weight. This is because none of your action is coming from that inspired space of being connected with yourself, instead it's coming from motivation, from outside of yourself without any understanding and appreciation of where you are, physically or emotionally.

Conversely, when you do like U, you are connected, more aligned with yourself and therefore instinctively take actions that nourish and support you. Instead of running flat out on the treadmill you decide to go a little easier, listening to your body and what feels good each day, depending on your energy levels, and you actually enjoy it. Your body is much more likely to lighten up with this inspired action, regardless of calorie input and output, rather than the motivated action because there is a whole lot more love and intelligence in the inspiration than the motivation. Love is what helps the world to go around and it definitely gets the light energy flowing freely through your body.

These three relationships - with food, your body and U, are The Holy Trinity of your BeUtiful body and they all need to be love-filled if you are wanting to transform your body. Let's work our way through each one of these relationships now and rekindle the love in them.

Part 2 - You and Food

The relationship between you and food ultimately determines the effect food will have on your weight, health and wellbeing. This special relationship is based upon three factors; your belief about that food, how you feel about eating it and how well your body digests it.

In The Name of Food

Throughout modern history we have become increasingly detached from the food we put into our body. Mass farming and manufacturing processes are squeezing the quality out of food and replacing it with cheaper, manmade ingredients to keep up with the ever increasing volume demands and commercial constraints. Food is business, first and foremost, and more often than not, decisions about the ingredients that go into food products are made from the perspective of profit rather than quality, health or, in the case of mass farmed live stock, morality.

We no longer eat to nourish our body, we eat fast, on-the-go, without even tasting food, let alone appreciating and enjoying it. Sometimes we even use food as a tool of self-harm, over-eating or under-eating, often with foods that damage our health because they're the most readily available options. It's not just the poor quality foods themselves causing the harm, our lack of thought and care for our body, that's allowing us to make these decisions, speaks volumes.

The problem is we're not biologically designed to tolerate this type of 'unconscious eating'. Just take our consumption of sugar alone, this has trebled since the 1960's according to 'Sugar Economics: How Sweet It Isn't', a report compiled by Morgan Stanley and published in 2015, supporting earlier claims published in the American Journal of Clinical Nutrition that we are consuming more sugar these days than our bodies are equipped to handle, leading to metabolic syndrome, obesity, kidney and cardiovascular disease. Not to mention the impact on your mood of consuming high amounts of sugar.

The way we eat today is practically unrecognisable from how our ancestors ate, but biologically we are not that different. It's no surprise then that we experience more illness and disease now, than we ever have in our history, ironic given the medical advancements and technology we have at our disposal. According to The National Cancer Institute, cancer is among the leading causes of death worldwide. In 2012, there were 14 million new cases and 8.2 million cancer-related deaths worldwide and the number of new cancer cases will rise to 22 million within the next two decades.

Food and lifestyle have been proven to be instrumental in that statistic and the following foods are considered among the most dangerous for health. What is most concerning is that they form the majority of the standard Western diet and are consumed daily, by adults and children as staples. When you start connecting the dots between food quality and the health of a population it is outrageous that they are continuing to be produced, marketed and sold without any restriction and health warnings on the labels. It makes you wonder who is benefitting from these trends in food consumption and disease, and if their intentions really are for the greater good and the health of a nation.

I don't want to fear anyone into making new choices but knowledge is power - here are the ten most dangerous foods for your health, as agreed by multiple nutrition based sources:

Meat and Processed Meats

Mass farmed livestock are pumped full of antibiotics and hormones, and reared in conditions that no living thing should be subjected to. Forget whether you think eating meat is OK or not from a moral perspective, that's your call and for each of us to decide what we are comfortable with. But, farmed in the way these animals are, a far cry from organic free-range livestock, no good can ever come from something so categorically wrong. For the welfare of the animal, the environment, surrounding communities and for the health of the end consumer, who's basically ingesting the hormone and pharmaceutical cocktail these animals are given on a daily basis.

When you eat this it causes digestive chaos because your body can't break it down, so the meat gets impacted on your intestinal walls creating a wrath of health issues from indigestion to high blood pressure and cancer. The meat sits in your system and putrefies, literally poisoning you from the inside out. Deli meats take this to a whole new level as they're exceptionally high in nitrates and sodium that are incredibly harmful to your health. The American Institute for

Cancer Research states that consumption of these meats is related to an increased risk of colon cancer. Nitrates are converted into nitrites which can form nitrosamines in your body and these are noted as a powerful cancer causing chemical.

Trans and Hydrogenated Fats

These fats are linked to increased risks of heart attack, stroke, cholesterol and diabetes, just to name but a few of the worlds biggest killers! Trans fatty acids are formed when manufacturers turn liquid oils into solid fats via a process called hydrogenation. Basically this messes with the fats atomic structure.

They're typically found in margarines, fried foods and baked goods like crackers. In fact, it is estimated that trans fats are found in 40% of food products in the supermarket[10], basically because they help food last longer. Eating even minimal amounts of trans fats is linked to a greater increase in cardiovascular disease according to a report published by Science Daily.

Trans fats raise your cholesterol and damage the walls of blood vessels, whilst putting your system under immense stress, particularly harming your liver. Always check your food labels and avoid all foods with trans fats. Even governments are taking this one seriously with The U.S. Food and Drug Administration approving a nationwide ban on partially hydrogenated oil in foods, which effectively will eliminate dietary trans fat when it goes into effect in 2018.

Refined Sugar

John Yudkin was a British professor of nutrition who had raised the alarm on sugar in 1972, in a book called Pure, White, and Deadly, stating "if only a small fraction of what we know about the effects of sugar were to be revealed in relation to any other material used as a food additive, that material would promptly be banned." At the time Yudkin was largely discredited by the food industry and his career suffered. However, he was right, and today's research proves it! A significant cause of obesity and diabetes according to the American Health Association, it also puts stress upon the pancreas, liver and digestive system.

Also, the nervous system is said to be compromised by up to 50 percent every time you eat sugar. This is bad news for your health as it makes you more susceptible to colds, flu, depression, hormonal imbalance, stress and weight gain. More recently, American doctor Robert Lustig, called for laws that restrict sugar as if it were tobacco due to its dangerous effect on our health. Remember, not all sugar is equal, natural sugars in fruits and honey are fine.

White Flour

It may seem relatively harmless but inside your body it behaves in much the same way as white sugar, putting huge stress on the pancreas and disrupting insulin levels.

In addition, highly processed white flour is missing the two most nutritious and fibre rich parts of the seed. A diet that consists of daily white flour, or white flour products, will leave you malnourished, constipated and vulnerable to chronic illness. Eating white flour literally compromises your system making you weaker.

It's all the processing that's the problem, not necessarily the grain itself. Although many people suffer with wheat intolerances, manifesting in a whole host of digestive issues, so you really do need to pay attention to how your body responds to eating wholegrain wheat foods if you still choose to. Also keep in mind that wheat has been mass farmed and hybridized to such an extent, with a cocktail of chemicals and fertilizers, you're not longer just eating a grain the way nature intended.

Pasteurized Milk

A bone of contention amongst many as we are encouraged to drink milk for stronger bones but according to nutritionist and author Patrick Holford, as we age we lose the ability to digest lactose which is a major component of milk, as a result it disrupts our digestion, causes bloating, food intolerances, inflammatory responses and acid. If your body is too acidic, this will weaken bones as your body will actually leach alkali minerals, like calcium and magnesium, from your bones and muscles to neutralize the excess acid.

Also, in countries where cow milk consumption is low, so is the rate of osteoporosis. However, in countries where cow milk is consumed daily, osteoporosis rates are the highest in the world. Milk does not make your bones stronger, it is a poor source of calcium because your body can't absorb it in the ratio with magnesium that is present in cow milk.

Most disturbing is the way milk is treated with heat, hormones, chemicals, preservatives and antibiotics, that all create toxicity in the body. That bowl of cereals every morning is not looking quite so innocent now with the white sugar, flour and milk poured on top! The most dangerous foods are those hiding in plain sight that we eat daily. And anyway, should we be consuming the milk of another animal, meant for its babies?

Fast Food

The fastest thing about fast food is the deterioration of your health because they literally contain no quality 'real food' ingredients. Fast food is full, however, of most of the previous mentioned most dangerous foods, and is really high in sodium to compound the negative impact of all the other health harming ingredients.

This is a deadly combination, this is not an exaggeration, and one that will reduce your life expectancy, remember the documentary Super-Size Me? Eating fast food every day for every meal is an extreme case, but, in less than a month the researchers health deteriorated that rapidly his doctors were seriously concerned for his wellbeing.

The US Department of Health and Human Services reported that the combination of poor diet and lack of physical activity causes 310,000 to 580,000 deaths every year, the types of foods that lead to these deaths are high in saturated fat, sodium and sugar, this is fast food!

Sodas and Diet Sodas

There are absolutely no nutrients that nourish your body found in soda. Your body does not gain anything from them nutritionally speaking, only stress, because they fill your system full of chemicals and sugar that deplete your body of nutrients.

A study published in the Cancer Epidemiology, Biomarkers and Prevention journal stated that drinking just two soda's per week can nearly double a person's risk of pancreatic cancer. Whilst Dr. Joseph Mercola says there "is 10 teaspoons of sugar" in just one can of soda and "30 to 55 mg of caffeine, artificial food colours and sulphites."

It also creates acid in the body which ultimately weakens bones, depletes vital mineral stores and makes you more susceptible to bacteria, infection and cancer, all of which can only survive if your body is acidic.

Doughnuts

Containing the rather 'unholy trinity' of the unhealthiest ingredients - white sugar, white flour and trans fat, these innocent enough looking rings of sweetness are not so sweet for your health. This is a lethal combination not just for your waist line but for all your major bodily systems. For instance, consumption of trans fat and sugar has been linked with a significantly higher risk of heart disease and diabetes.

Before you get too sad, there are incredible donut alternatives that are made with wholesome, plant based ingredients. Don't knock them until you've tried them!

Potato Chips

Its not really the fault of the potato, but when foods are fried at high temperatures they can form acrylamide which is a known carcinogen.

Not only are chips high in fat they are often coated with salt making them extremely high in sodium and this raises blood pressure and cholesterol and ultimately increases your risk of heart attack and stroke.

Also, a study published in Cancer Science in 2005 linked a high salt diet with increased gastric cancer.

Canned Soups

When you see canned foods you are looking at a stock pile of salt! Chicken soup for the soul maybe, but with this amount of sodium your body suffers significantly. In what is considered perhaps a 'healthy' food choice, some cans of soup can contain as much as 890 milligrams of sodium which translates to nearly your full day's quota.

In excess, sodium causes the body to retain water, and disrupts the delicate ratio between the other alkali minerals - calcium, potassium and magnesium. This puts tremendous stress on your cells, and causes your blood pressure to sky rocket if it isn't corrected, and significantly increases your risk of heart attack and stroke. According to the American Health Association 97 percent of American children consume too much sodium and it can lead to serious organ damage.

Redefining Food

What we eat has changed drastically from 50 years ago, food has become increasingly varied over time, which has its benefits, but a lot these foods have been 'made' rather than 'grown'.

The challenge is that we have collectively grouped all foods and food products as equals - they are not. Natural, fresh, organic fruits, vegetables, nuts, seeds and whole grains, for example, are not the same as processed diet foods, low fat foods, fast foods and food products with e-numbers, chemicals, and additives in them.

The problem is that we are eating all of this 'food' and we are getting heavier, feeling tired, eating larger portions, developing hormonal imbalances and experiencing a range of health and wellbeing challenges.

In today's world of food, it is no longer just our medicine but it can be our poison, too. Knowing the difference is the choice between feeling light or heavy, experiencing ease or dis-ease.

We need to be more precise about what food actually is because then we can begin to address our relationship with it from a solid foundation that is conducive to the way nature intended and where real food is not the diet enemy, it is the solution!

What do you have on your plate? Has it been grown, reared even, or has it been processed in a food factory?

The latter your body mostly has no idea what to do with, it gets stored and then creates stress on your system. The amount of 'diet foods' that are full of chemical sweeteners and altered fats is scary, as is the effect this has on your body. Yet, so many people are eating them, because they're low calorie, and wondering why their body is finding it difficult to feel satisfied, find balance and feel light.

With natural food, your body knows how to process it. Your body is genius at digesting - absorbing the good stuff and getting rid of what it doesn't need. However, if you eat something that your body can't digest, then you have a problem, your body literally can't process it. Those foods start to accumulate, slowing your entire digestive system down in the process.

I know nutritionists haven't always got the 'cool factor' around the dinner table, but, by natural food I'm not just talking celery sticks and lettuce leaves. I'm talking about the foods that are a pleasure to eat, foods that feel good to eat, are delicious, comforting, and most importantly, your body can digest. Think whole-food ingredients, high quality, pure foods, free from preservatives, additives and all sorts of other unnatural ingredients masquerading as food. Cakes made with gluten-free flours and sweetened with honey instead of chemical sweeteners, blueberry buckwheat pancakes with real maple syrup and berries and indulgent raw chocolate bars with whole coconut milk instead of hormone-fed cow milk.

If you could acquaint yourself with this kind of food, and disregard the rest, then the pleasure and medicinal nature of eating would go hand-in-hand, as nature intended.

Remember the list of the ten most harmful foods for your health? Let's contrast this with the ten healthiest foods and you will see exactly what I mean by 'real food' as opposed to manufactured food products.

This list is compiled from a selection of sources from the USA and Europe, including nutritionists and dietician's published in Medical News Today and Forbes Magazine. Notice that all ten are plant based:

Avocados

They provide up to twenty different nutrients including essential fatty acids, fibre, minerals, vitamins, antioxidants and folic acid. They alkalize the body and act as a nutrient booster helping the body absorb fat soluble nutrients.

Almonds

These nuts are full of minerals and vitamin E proving to be highly effective heart protectors, blood pressure and cholesterol reducers and metabolism boosters. In just one ounce you will get 12 percent of your daily protein, 35 percent of your daily vitamin E, and as much calcium as in 1/4 cup of milk.

Broccoli

Research suggests broccoli has potent anti-cancer properties and phytonutrients that reduce the risk of developing heart disease, strokes and diabetes. In just 100g of broccoli you will eat 150 percent of your daily vitamin C. B vitamins, minerals, dietary fibre and antioxidants all combine to make broccoli a powerhouse of nutrition.

Berries (blueberries, goji berries, raspberries)

The rich colours of berries reflect the array of potent antioxidants they contain which are very powerful health protectors, healers and cell repairers. Berries are incredibly anti-ageing, they preserve brain and memory function, can help lower blood pressure and blueberries specifically have been associated with helping to control body weight.

Chia Seeds

These tiny seeds are packed with essential omega 3, fibre, vitamins, minerals, protein and antioxidants. They provide a wide spectrum of nutrients giving the body an extreme boost in health and vitality. The omega 3 protects the heart, joints and brain function, it stimulates the metabolism, reduces inflammation and helps lower cholesterol.

Dark Chocolate

Perhaps the richest source of magnesium on the planet, extremely alkali and full of antioxidants, this makes cacao one of the most nutrient dense foods in the world. Its nutrients help to balance blood sugar and control appetite whilst protecting the heart and reducing your risk of heart attack. It boosts your mood and gives you that feel good factor which makes life a little sweeter!

Leafy Greens (kale and spinach etc.)

Minerals, and lots of them, especially magnesium, iron and calcium, all essential for your health and wellbeing. Iron boosts your blood and energy whilst magnesium and calcium strengthens bones, neutralizes acid, reduces inflammation and heat, soothes the heart and nervous system and balances blood sugar.

Seaweeds

One of the richest sources of iodine which is essential for the proper functioning of the thyroid gland and the entire endocrine system. Seaweeds are also incredibly rich in minerals and antioxidants that are among the best protectors of health and have great levels of vitamin D, which is vital for the absorption of calcium and bone health.

Apples

An apple a day certainly does keep the doctor away with an excellent provision of pectin, a soluble fibre that can lower cholesterol. They also contain quercetin that has anti-inflammatory properties, can help reduce allergies, especially hay fever and they may help prevent respiratory problems.

Beans

Beans mean fibre and this means digestive health, a happy colon and bowel, easier weight management and efficient elimination of waste. They are also a diabetic's best friend as they help balance blood sugar, they also provide high quality protein that is easily absorbed by your body.

Having said all of this, food comes to life in your body, so there really are no universally 'healthy' foods because we are all so different. One persons poison will be a vitamin for somebody else, and this is important to remember, because there is nothing intelligent, or inspired, about mindlessly eating a raw vegan diet, for example, without being conscious of how your body is responding.

The Power of Food

Food does have an effect on your physical body, but it isn't just the food itself that's making an impact. How you feel about food, your intention for eating, how you feel about your body, and what your thoughts and beliefs are around food, you health and weight are all part of the equation.

To add to this, food will not just effect your physical body, it will also affect how you feel, which in turn will impact your physical wellbeing.

Food and emotions are inseparable. What you eat effects how you feel, therefore you must consider your eating within a holistic framework, encompassing this greater understanding. So many diets are oblivious to the impact food has on your emotional and mental state, so it's not surprising they don't work.

Let's delve a little deeper into the power of food.

The Physical Power of Food

Vitamins, minerals, antioxidants, enzymes, amino acids, essential fatty acids - all of these are nutrients that are essential for our survival and they are all found in food. Food also provides intelligence, which informs each cell in your body, instructing the vast myriad of functions and systems to synergistically collaborate the precise conditions for your continued thriving.

Food has a purpose. We are not meant to simply eat for the sake of eating, we are designed to eat real food that has been designed to be eaten! Everything that we need to live healthy lives in BeUtiful bodies is right here for us, waiting to be eaten! Sweet potatoes don't just grow for the sake of growing, they play a vital role, like every other natural food, in providing the nutrients for life, and intelligence that is waiting to be transformed in your body into something BeUtiful.

Did you know that walnuts lower cholesterol? Avocados balance female hormones, coconut raises your metabolism and helps to encourage lightness as do almonds. Celery is fabulous for strengthening bones, potatoes are natures Prozac, mung beans are excellent for reducing cellulite, flaxseeds can help reduce high blood pressure as can hawthorn berries, turmeric is a powerful anti-inflammatory, ginger aids digestion, and cherries get rid of gout.

Also, our body carries out millions of processes, all of which require energy and nutrients found in food. Some of those essential nutrients are needed to stabilize the central nervous system, boost liver and kidney function, to nourish our brain and to help our body cope with stress whilst boosting happy mood hormones.

In nutrition talk, at least, happiness comes in the form of sufficient amounts of omega 3, B vitamins, tryptophan, magnesium and chromium. In food terms this looks like omega 3 rich walnuts, avocado, chia, flax and pumpkin seeds. Sunflower seeds, quinoa, rice, fresh fruits and vegetables that are full of B vitamins, with beans and mint leaves that are rich in tryptophan, raw cacao and leafy greens for magnesium and almonds, bananas and even more leafy greens for chromium.

Together, these foods help maintain balanced brain chemistry and hormone activity to help you stay feeling happy and positive. If you are not eating these nutrients then your physical body is not getting the ingredients it needs to support these functions.

Omega 3 is also essential for a healthy metabolism and feeling light. If you don't have enough of this essential fatty acid you are literally trapping the fat into your cells as your cell walls become less flexible and diffusion from cell to cell becomes difficult. As fat is dense, it gets trapped inside the cell and losing it becomes nearly impossible if your cell walls aren't permeable.

You can always tell when someone has recently 'dieted' by counting calories as a means to lose weight rather than feeding their body to allow it to release excess weight naturally. They lose weight on their faces, and for women on their breasts, but the stubborn areas stay stuck. If you have stubborn areas of fat, I suggest you start sprinkling ground flaxseed or chia seeds on your breakfast and snack on pumpkin seeds! Better yet, hemp seeds, with a perfect ratio of omega's and amino acids, they have incredible health benefits. You can buy them from most health stores.

Having said all of this, there is no point in over-thinking your diet in the fear not getting all the nutrients, in exactly the right amounts and in exactly the right ratios to one another. For a start, who really knows what the optimum amount of these nutrients are, as we are all so different and have very different nutritional needs, depending on what's going on in our lives.

Going to the other extreme of stuffing yourself full of all the vitamins, minerals, antioxidants, lotions, potions and superfoods that you can get your hands on is not going to do you any good either. Many of us fall into this trap of feeling like we need every known supplement and start popping pills left, right, and center! There was a time when my supplement drawer began to take over my whole kitchen.

Relax and breathe. Whilst we are trying to nurture more awareness around food in a positive way and feed your body the nutrients that it needs to facilitate your BeUtiful body, we don't need to get into this micro managing situation with food either, grabbing at every superfood in sight is not an intelligent way to feed your body.

The Emotional Power of Food

Food contains emotional nutritional components, and what you eat directly effects how you feel. The challenge, however, is that as soon as we start talking about emotions and feelings, things can appear to be getting 'hairy fairy', requiring a 'leap of faith' as something to believe in rather than a logical, measurable process rooted in tangible components. Thanks to biology, epigenetic's and an understanding of the vibrational nature of the Universe, the latter is now the case. Food does effect how you feel, and this is how:

The Vagus Nerve

"There is a superhighway between the brain and GI system that holds great sway over humans."[11] A significant part of that 'highway', is the Vagus Nerve, with information flowing directly between the brain and the stomach, in both directions. What happens in your brain directly effects your stomach and what happens in your stomach directly effects your brain. Therefore, what you eat and how well it gets digested directly effects your mood, specifically as a result of your microbiome. There are "10-100 trillion symbiotic microbial cells harbored by each person, primarily bacteria in the gut"[12] the human microbiome is basically the genes that these bacteria cells harbor. Research is now strongly indicating that the microbiome "can activate the vagus nerve and that such activation plays a critical role in mediating effects on the brain and behaviour," and "understanding the induction and transmission of signals in the vagus nerve may have important implications for the development of microbial or nutrition based therapeutic strategies for mood disorders."[13]

The Second Brain

The digestive system has its own nervous system that communicates with the rest of the body using information gathered through the intestinal vili, the finger like projections within the intestinal walls. In this sense, the digestive system is referred to as the 'second brain' and responsible for that 'gut feeling'. This "mind-gut connection is not just metaphorical. Our brain and gut are connected by an extensive network of neurons and a highway of chemicals and hormones that constantly provide feedback about how hungry we are, whether or not we're experiencing stress, or if we've ingested a disease-causing microbe. This information superhighway is called the brain-gut axis and it provides constant updates on the state of affairs at your two ends,"[14] directly influencing your brain chemistry and mood.

Hormone Production

Hormones are chemical messengers that directly influence your state of health, weight, energy and mood. Serotonin, cortisol, insulin, dopamine, estrogen and testosterone, all of which are affected by how you eat and what you eat. For example, serotonin is released within your digestive system, if there are digestive disturbances, like food allergies or intolerances, then this directly impacts the release of serotonin, the happy hormone, and your mood will suffer. If you skip meals your insulin and cortisol levels will be negatively effected, this will also directly effect how you feel. With hormones, it isn't just each one that is important, but the ratio between them all, this delicate balance is extremely influenced by food. Also, there are amino acids required from food to facilitate the synthesis of certain hormones, if you don't eat enough of the right foods your hormones will suffer, and so will your mood.

Blood Sugar

"Controlling your blood sugar levels is absolutely critical to controlling your mood, energy, and motivation. If you've ever known someone who is "Jekyll and Hyde", there is a very good chance that they are constantly riding what is commonly referred to as the Blood Sugar Rollercoaster."[15] This is one of my favorite explanations of the impact of blood sugar on how you feel. This is common knowledge but too often we forget to connect the dots between what we've eaten and how we feel. "Your blood sugar level is determined by the carbs that you eat. Eating the wrong type of carbs will send you for a ride on the rollercoaster. Eating the right type of carb will keep you safely off the rollercoaster, allowing you to have happy, energetic, and fun moods."[16] I have worked with so many clients that feel depressed and irritable, thinking there is 'something wrong' with them, when in reality, there is nothing wrong, it's just that their blood sugar is fluctuating so wildly, from a state of high alert to exhaustion, from the innocent enough looking coffee and cake, that they can't find their balance. By the way, caffeine and sugar is a lethal combination if you are anywhere near sensitive to sugar. Don't mix these two if you want to maintain some semblance of yourself!

Tryptophan

This is an essential amino acid that is needed for normal growth and development, along with balancing your circadian rhythm, it is a key ingredient in making serotonin, the good mood hormone. Tryptophan "acts like a natural mood regulator, since it has the ability to help the body produce and balance certain hormones naturally. Supplementing with tryptophan-rich foods or taking supplements helps bring on natural calming effects, induces sleep, fights anxiety and can also help burn more body fat. Tryptophan has also been found to stimulate the release of growth hormones and even reduce food cravings for carbohydrates and help kick a sugar addiction in some cases."[17] Tryptophan rich foods include spirulina, bananas, seeds, nuts, oats, brown rice, quinoa, beans, legumes and mint leaves.

So, why is this important? Because your physical state is a direct result, or manifestation, of your mental and emotional state. Think about that for a moment. If your mental and emotional state 'causes' your physical state, why are we just concerned with eating to 'fix' our physical body? Surely a much quicker and more effective approach would be to positively address our mental and emotional state through food and lifestyle too, integrating this more complete understanding of how our body works.

So remember, when you are feeling negative or depressed, it may not be external circumstances to blame. In fact, your depression could be the destabilizing effect of eating a food that doesn't feel good for your body.

Sometimes s*** happens. Of course, you feel the effect of that, but if you find yourself feeling generally down or susceptible to mood and energy swings, then your food could be the issue. The beauty is, if you are conscious of it and make a different choice, food could also be your solution.

You may think, "I'm drinking too much coffee, what if I just had one a day and didn't add the sugar because maybe this is creating a roller coaster of emotion making me feel stressed and anxious?" Or, "what if I stopped skipping lunch? Maybe my blood sugar levels would stabilize and this would help lift my mood as my body's energy would feel more supported and grounded."

The Vibrational Power of Food

This Universe is energy based. Our body is energy, everything around us is energy. Thoughts and emotions are energy. Food is also vibrational energy.

Back in the 1930's and 40's, an expert in electromagnetism, French scientist and researcher, André Simoneton, created an experiment that measured the electromagnetic waves, or vibration, of foods and the human body. Firstly, he found that for good health a human must maintain a vibration of 6500 angstrom, a metric used to express wavelengths of visible light. He then went on to rate foods by their vibration and categorized them, ranging from the highest category, measuring between 6,500 and 10,000 angstrom, which included: fresh fruits, vegetables, olives, sweet almonds, sunflower seeds, coconut, soy, peanuts, hazelnuts and whole grains. In the case of soy and whole grains remember this was pre GMO and chemical hybridization. To the lowest category, registering practically no measurement of angstrom, consisting of margarine, conserves, alcoholic spirits, refined white sugar and bleached flour.

This vibrational energy doesn't just interact with your physical body, it also interacts with your mental and emotional state, directly influencing how you feel. Thoughts and emotions are measurable vibrational energy too, with positive emotions, like unconditional love and appreciation, being equivalent to the highest frequencies, and fear to the lowest, similar to that of the margarine, alcoholic spirits, refined white sugar and bleached flour. You are what you eat!

Generally speaking, the higher our vibrational energetic state, the more healthy, alive and conscious you feel. Meditation, for example, raises your vibrational energetic state and this is why it has so many healing benefits.

A lower vibrational energy means that the energy wave is much slower in frequency. This 'lower' state is more conducive to illness and diseases, along with a more negative emotional state and mental process, making it more difficult for you to connect with your inner being and guidance. Lower vibrational energy is 'heavier,' often weighing down your thoughts, emotions, and physical body.

In practice, and for your comfort, a high vibrational energy paired with a sense of grounded stability in your body and emotional state, creates a beautiful balance between sensitivity without it being overwhelming.

If food is energy and we are energy, when we eat, the energy vibration of the food will interact and effect the energy vibration of our body. We are what we eat, physically and energetically.

Natural foods are usually high vibrational foods, with raw food and sprouts being among the highest, whilst cooked food and animal products have a lower vibration. Junk foods, and those with additives and chemicals, are at the lowest end of the energy spectrum.

It's important to understand that 'high' does not necessarily mean 'good', and 'low' does not necessarily mean 'bad'. Remember, we are always trying to bring you closer to a balanced, more comfortable state. If you are in a sensitized state of anxiousness or stress, a raw salad with superfood sprouts is not going to help you feel any calmer, it will exacerbate your sensitivity.

If you eat low vibrational foods all of the time then you're starving yourself of vital life force energy so you will feel 'low', your thinking will be more susceptible to negativity and your body will be effected by this too. These foods clog your energy pathways and allow for accumulation, emotionally and physically. Forget feeling inspired to get out and walk or get on your yoga mat under these conditions, it's an uphill battle requiring some serious willpower as you feel like you are literally dragging yourself around. If this sounds like you then stop trying to muster more willpower and beating yourself up about it. Stop, take a moment, look through your food, and see where you can start eating more vital life force energy.

Conversely, if you eat high vibrational foods, full of vital life force energy, then you are more likely to feel positive emotions. You will feel much clearer as these foods detoxify and cleanse your system, leaving your mood feeling light and your thinking positive. This will translate into a light feeling, energized, healthy, toxin free body.

By understanding the power of food at this level, we are creating a new platform to make inspired decisions about what we want to eat, making more intelligent and meaningful choices that serve our wellbeing.

What's On Your Plate?

Understanding the physical, emotional and vibrational power of food, now take a look at what's on your plate. Is it nutrient rich or poor, fresh or processed, natural or toxic, nourishment or restriction, light or heaviness, peace or stress, pleasure or guilt, alive or dead?

Tonight, before you go to bed write in your BeUtiful Body journal the food you have eaten today and ask yourself:

» *What did you put on your plate today?*

» *What kind of energy was in your food?*

» *What are you actually feeding yourself, physically, emotionally and vibrationally?*

I'm not asking you to quantify what's on your plate in calorific terms, I want you to become conscious of what is really on your plate, appreciating the power of food, on all levels, what it actually contains, beyond calories, its ability to effect you physically, emotionally, mentally and energetically.

Seeing beyond the mainstream diet approach to food will help you to unravel your own relationship with food and understand what is really going on, and how food is effecting your unique body. It will also help you to simplify your emotional connection with food, weeding out the more negative fear based beliefs and streamlining the entire eating process with more love, for food and for yourself.

Expanding your awareness about food, to accommodate this broader more accurate understanding of food and nutrition, will help naturally inspire different thoughts and behaviour with food without you having to be told do this and eat that. The more aware you are, the more you can make inspired choices and feel empowered within your relationship with food.

Different thinking, different behavior, different results!

Eating Consciously

Eating consciously is something we have forgotten to do, but it isn't a new idea. As a species, we would have never survived if we didn't eat consciously. Not paying attention when eating a certain plant or berry caused us to feel ill, or even worse, caused our death. If humans hadn't made the connection between food and health then we wouldn't have survived on this planet. The fact that we ate consciously allowed us to learn what was good for us, and what wasn't and to eat accordingly. Otherwise it could have been extinction by too many lethal berry combinations!

If we choose to find the space and create time to do so, conscious eating is our most natural and instinctive way of eating. We have so many issues with eating, unhealthy relationships with food, and heavy feeling bodies because we have not been eating consciously. If we were conscious, we would have figured out long ago what feels good and what doesn't, what creates more balance and what takes us further away from it, what creates lightness and what makes us feel like we are going to burst out of our skinny jeans! The best part, we would have acted upon that wisdom instead of being totally disempowered and confused by trying to keep up with the latest diet and what everyone else thinks we 'should' be eating to lose weight.

It is not surprising that we blame food. Food definitely felt like the enemy, but the only enemy I had was myself, it was me making unconscious choices that didn't feel good for my body, it was me that continually ignored my body, it was me that thought thoughts and felt feelings that harmed my body, and it was me that ate foods that didn't feel good and in ways that created heaviness, either in my head or sometimes physically in my body, too. I was in too deep to realize that if I felt heavy and bloated, even if I had only ate a salad, then I was eating food that my body didn't like in ways that were not loving.

So now you must become conscious of what is actually going on in your body, outside of the diet drama and nutrition text books. Once you get 'conscious' you can take your eating to another level and become an intuitive eater. Not only is this the best way to eat and nourish your body, it is the only way to eat as an expression of self-love, and, it is all about the love, because love is light!

To keep things simple, I have broken the intuitive eating process down into three parts: before, during and after eating! The next time you eat I want you to engage in the following process, with your BeUtiful Body journal right beside you, so you can experience this level of conscious awareness around food and begin to eat intuitively.

Before Eating

Your body needs nutrients from food to function, so at some point it will let you know this. Hunger is not bad, remind yourself not to be irritated that you are hungry, it means you are alive, surely that's a good thing!

Our basic purpose for eating is to give the body exactly the right tools to function optimally. For example, to have harmonious hormones, a comfortable blood pressure, energy for metabolism, fuel for brain function and proper digestion. If we don't eat the foods our body needs, then all of these things suffer. We feel the results; illness, disease, stress, lethargy, discomfort, and heaviness.

We can be emotionally hungry for food too. Are you hungry for food or are you hungry for emotional nourishment? Ask the question, feel the answer, and do not ignore yourself.

If it's the latter then I always begin with getting a drink, usually something warm because it's more comforting than cold, like a hot chocolate made with cacao, almond milk and honey. Then take a few moments whilst you sip your warm comforting drink and consider how you can emotionally nourish yourself with what you feel you need in this moment. Once you know then take the action, maybe it's a call to your best friend, watching your favourite movie, having a bubble bath, getting yourself to a yoga class, or whatever it is that you feel will feed you emotionally. Often giving yourself this level of attention is good enough to inspire the most appropriate next step.

If you are hungry for food then now is the time to tune into what your body is hungry for. Don't ignore or suppress, instead, feed your body exactly what it needs.

Raw or cooked, cold or warm, a snack or something more substantial? Do you feel you need energy, do you feel like you need strength, do you want to feel calmer, or do you want to feel energized? How you answer these questions will begin to inspire your decisions about what to eat in a way that best serves your body.

Don't worry too much about making the wrong choice. There is no wrong choice, only an opportunity to begin to figure out what different feelings and foods mean for your body. When reading food labels stay focused on the ingredients list, rather than the numbers, to inspire your choices.

As you heal your relationship with food, you find it increasingly easier to be aware of your hunger and find more comfort in fulfilling your body's needs. Recognizing when your body is hungry and needing food is the first crucial part of being a conscious eater and will allow you the freedom to consider what it is you are really hungry for.

When you have a sad relationship with food, you never even gift yourself the luxury of a choice. You simply eat either whatever is in your path, or as little as you can get away with. This will leave you feeling dissatisfied and irritated.

Also, when you have anxiety around the thought of eating, and you try to put it off, this sends anxiety ridden messages to your body and you begin to feel stressed and tired. When your body switches over to this mode, achieving a light feeling body is impossible as your body moves to survival and storage in an attempt to protect itself, from you!

Learning to listen to your body is so powerful. It sends a message that you are willing to care for yourself rather than ignoring your needs. Most dis-ease today is born out of ignoring your needs, which produces more negative behavior that doesn't allow your BeUtiful body because you're totally out of balance, and out of alignment with yourself.

Being aware of your need for food and paying attention to it is an excellent step toward conscious eating and nurturing a powerful intention to nourish your body. Ask yourself again, "are you feeling good about what you are about to eat?"

During Your Meal

Now you are eating, mid mouthful of yummy food, ask yourself these questions and be ready to note down any insights in your BeUtiful Body journal:

» *How are you feeling?*

» *Do you like the taste of the food?*

» *Does it feel good to be eating this?*

» *Is it hitting the spot?*

Consciously eating is about directing thought, and energy follows thought, toward how your body is relating to this food, in this moment, and vice versa. Put in another way, it is how well you are digesting this food, or rather, what type of relationship is your body having with this food. Essentially, digestion is key for a light feeling body, and digestion is the result of the relationship between food and your body, and you need to create the environment that allows your body to have the best chance at easily digesting food in peace.

If your food choice isn't a happy feeling relationship with your body, for example, you're not enjoying the taste or eating doesn't feel that pleasurable, don't worry, this is vital information and an opportunity to inspire your next meal with what not to eat. In this way you are literally building your own nutrition manual relative to your body and U.

A common behaviour around food, especially when under the influence of diet mentality, is to get eating over and done with as quickly as possible to avoid the 'problem'. When you eat like this it's usually super fast, almost inhaled, with the lowest calorie food you could get your hands on at the time and you still feel guilty about having to eat. You don't even chew the food properly and so your stomach is now filled with large chunks of food that it can't break-down, too much air from eating so fast and guilt. This is a problem. Physically, your body is unable to digest what you're eating so you feel heavy and uncomfortable, and this undigested food accumulates and becomes toxic. Mentally, if digestion is disturbed then so is your thinking and state of mind because of the direct link between your gut and your brain. Emotionally, you're not allowing yourself to receive the nourishment and pleasure of eating so you feel unfulfilled and your mood suffers as a direct consequence of the negative impact on your digestion and mental state. Most importantly however, this whole eating experience is completely devoid of self-love, the most vital nutrient of all, and if you didn't feel the love then you will still feel hungry!

It is so important that we find the time to gift ourselves with the space to embrace the physical and emotional nourishment from our food and allow the goodness to be absorbed. This is key in healing our relationship with food, making peace with eating and making peace with our body.

When we are conscious of eating in the moment, we are blessed with the awareness of all our senses being awake to how the food smells, tastes and feels. Now you are in a position to know if this food feels good to eat. If it does, then great! You are putting food into your body that it loves and so it will love you in return, contributing to your health, wellbeing and your BeUtiful body. But, if your food choice doesn't feel good then pay attention, your body is trying to tell you this food isn't nurturing the state of balance and nourishment that you need.

Eating should feel good and it should be pleasurable, anything else and you are not eating the right foods for you in this moment.

Conscious eating during meal times is simply asking the question, does what you are eating taste and feel good to eat? If yes, then you are on it! If no, stop, eat something else, or at least don't repeat this choice at your next meal.

After Eating

Your meal is over, you've finished eating, ask yourself these questions and write them down in your BeUtiful Body journal:

» *Did you enjoy your food?*

» *Do you still feel hungry, content, or like you've eaten too much?*

» *Do you feel comfortable or heavy in your stomach?*

An hour or two later, ask yourself these same questions to fully check-in with yourself. How has your body reacted, do you feel nourished and energetic, or do you feel heavy, bloated, and lethargic? It is important to be aware of how your body assimilates and digests certain foods.

You need to pay attention to these indicators because this is your body giving you feedback on what's good and what's not, relative to your unique body.

There is no golden rule that suits everyone, and this is why diets don't work. Everybody is different. To address the differences, we all need to become conscious of what works for us and this is achieved through conscious eating.

Do you feel happy about what you ate or do you feel guilty?

Pay attention to the emotional responses certain foods give. Food is energy and affects you on all levels. If you are feeling calm and content after eating then wonderful! But if you are feeling unsatisfied and anxious then maybe that food didn't serve you well.

Notice the dialogue running through your mind about what you have eaten, if you feel guilty then this is going to negatively impact the relationship between your body and the food you ate, and you'll feel it, perhaps through a bloated stomach.

It is amazing how many times we will eat the same lunch and not feel good and still fail to make the connection between how we feel and what we ate. Even worse, continue to eat the same thing day after day. Stop this self-harm!

How are you feeling? If you don't feel great then something needs to change, don't keep repeating the same old patterns. Asking the question, how do you feel, creates the space for a non-habitual, more inspired choice to be made.

Self-Love or Self-Harm?

Eating habits and behaviors around food give tremendous insight into a person, how they feel about their body, how they feel about themselves and how they feel about life. Forget sex, religion and politics, look at what you eat and how, this will tell you so much more about yourself!

Beliefs, thoughts, opinions and emotions, all get played out through food choices. Whether we care about food or not, if we are super strict or completely free reign, micro analyzing or controlling, trying to be 'good' but then never being 'good enough' with guilt infested 'cheat days,' or completely starving ourselves and then binge eating. The big thing to know is that none of this is actually about food, but it does say a lot about how you feel about yourself and if you are 'using' food as a tool for self-love or self-harm.

What you eat is like a mirror image of how you feel about your body and yourself, but it isn't just the food choice in itself that tells us this, it is the intention behind the choice that holds the most power and ultimately determines whether it is love or harm.

For example, if you eat fruit and vegetables, this doesn't automatically mean that you're loving yourself. You could be on vegetable juices all day, supposedly very healthy, but not everyone is doing this from a place of love for their body, believe me.

It isn't so much what you do, but why you do it. This is what your body is really listening and responding to. Your beliefs, emotions and intentions imbue the food you eat and ultimately determine how well it will be digested, if the goodness will be unlocked and absorbed by your body and if it will leave you feeling satisfied and content. You cannot eat celery sticks out of sheer restriction and diet mindedness, chew your way through them begrudgingly, and then expect your body to respond in kind. Hence, 'a little bit of what you fancy does you good'. An old wives tale maybe, but wise.

You have to get real about your intentions that inform your food choices. Are they coming from a place of loving your body, or are you wanting to punish, restrict and control because you're constantly body shaming yourself? Even if you think you don't give food that much thought, then perhaps you're not giving yourself the attention you need and deserve either.

Understanding what is underlying your relationship with food will help you to bring more conscious awareness to your choices, instead of just repeating the same patterns and getting the same results, regardless of the actual food you choose.

The magic isn't just in the blueberries, it's in your intention!

Eating For Comfort

Between our instinct to eat for comfort, which is undeniable, and the usual diet rules that say a big fat "no" to comfort eating because food is just fuel, this topic of emotional eating has become a point of enormous self-sabotage. It seems whenever food, comfort and pleasure get involved together, we are pre-programmed to feel guilty. So, if we do answer our body's request for comfort, then any comfort that is achieved is short lived, and quickly followed by a barrage of guilt, shame and last but not least, heaviness.

In and of itself, eating for comfort is a relatively logical solution to help yourself to feel better. After all, we're not robots, we do have an emotional relationship with food as it's essential for our survival. Also, when we eat, we have a physical, as well as an emotional, response to food.

The challenge is, that most often, when we feel in need of comfort, we don't feel very good, and therefore naturally, we are attracted to foods of a similar vibration to our emotional state, so here comes the low vibe fast food! We eat it, despite our belief that it's bad for us, ride the initial wave of feeling good, and then come crashing down as guilt and a refined carbohydrate coma take hold.

But what if we were able to choose slightly higher vibration foods that would also give us comfort? What if we raised our standards and instead of going straight for fast food, gave ourselves other options that hit the spot, on all levels, comforting in the short run, supporting in the long run and free from guilt?

I absolutely believe that comfort eating is not a bad thing in itself. This idea that we should just eat for fuel is robotic and completely underestimates the effect of food and its relationship with our body, not just our body's relationship with food. This is a two-way highway, with information flowing in both directions.

When you realize that you don't feel good and you seek comfort, why is that a bad thing to do? How you go about it certainly needs to be consciously considered, but the process is a healthy one. Why would you stay feeling bad when you could help yourself to feel better? And because food is vibration, emotion is vibration, thought is vibration, eating can be one way to help ourselves when done in an intelligent way. And we do need to eat three times a day, so why not factor in comfort inducing effects at one of those mealtimes?

Embracing all aspects of the power of food, whilst being aware of your body and emotional state is an incredible way to nourish your body. Don't shy away from this. I know every diet under the sun has told you comfort eating is 'bad' but how can working with yourself, being conscious of your emotions, actively wanting to feel good and then helping yourself to feel better be a bad thing?

If you eat a whole pizza then feel guilty as you're drowning in a cheesy haze, then yes, that was not really the definition of 'comfort', it has to last longer than an hour to count, and it certainly wasn't a love filled choice!

When something tastes good it will help you to feel better[18], but this is only part of the reason why you feel comforted after eating the usual go-to comfort foods like pizza, cakes and ice cream. "Carbohydrates set off a series of chemical reactions that ultimately lead to a boost in brain serotonin,"[19] and higher levels of serotonin mean that you will feel content and comforted. But this is short lived, because if you do eat fast food you are 51% more likely to experience depression than those who don't eat fast food, according to a paper by the University of Granada published in the Public Health Nutrition Journal.

Raise your standards and go for better quality comfort food, choose buckwheat rather than white pasta, baked sweet potato fries instead of regular fries, pizzas full of veggies rather than processed meat, dark or raw chocolate over cheap milk chocolate, raw desserts (the best thing about raw food are the desserts) instead of processed cakes, coconut based ice-cream instead of cow's milk ice-cream. Mindful, conscious, comfort eating.

One of my clients was a 16 year old girl, she was struggling with her weight, feeling very self-conscious of her body and under the pressure of her exams. Through no fault of her own, in fact, through her natural born instinct, she had discovered the comfort and pleasure to be found in food. She found temporary relief, comfort, even relaxation, but then felt so ashamed of herself and guilty for eating what she had.

All of this guilt and shame exasperated her negative body image and her body didn't know whether it was coming or going, neither did she. Her family, through concern of her wellbeing, became very watchful and judgmental of what she ate in an attempt to persuade her to eat healthier foods, which only made things worse, and peer pressure wasn't helping either.

This girl was in need of comfort, trying to make her stop eating for comfort was totally counterproductive, but, teaching her how to eat for comfort in a way that supported rather than sabotaged her was key. It turned her shame that she felt for herself into understanding, and that what she was doing wasn't crazy, and with just a little more information and understanding about the nature of food, and that we are meant to feel comforted by it, she was empowered to care and nourish herself in the best possible way. Experiencing all the comfort and balance, she was looking for, but without the guilt and negative effect on her body weight and health.

To transform your comfort eating into long-lasting comfort and pleasure, whilst still contributing to a healthy, light feeling body, practice these three principles daily, with every meal, and especially if you feel the impulse to eat for comfort:

» Don't Eat Beyond The Limits of Your Beliefs - There is never any comfort in eating foods you believe are either 'bad' for you, will make you heavy or damage your health in someway. Always make choices about food that are within your current belief system, especially when it comes to seeking more comfort and balance. In the meantime, challenge your beliefs and then experiment as you are able to factor in all aspects that effect your state of health, weight and wellbeing, as we've been discussing.

» Focus on Quality - The most enduring comfort will always be found in foods that are quality rich and made with loving attention to detail. There is a vast nutritional and energetic difference between poor quality mass produced foods and high quality handmade foods. You can taste the difference, if you're paying attention, and your body will feel the difference too. Always focus on quality and choose foods that are befitting your body, don't allow your standards to drop, even when you're not feeling good enough!

» Allow Yourself to Receive - Many of us are more comfortable 'giving' than 'receiving', but to feel nourished and comforted we have to open ourselves up to receiving the nutrition and support within food and allow ourselves to experience pleasure, without guilt. The more we are open to receiving, the better the food will get digested and the nutrients will be easily absorbed deep within the body. If we don't, food won't get digested well, the nutrients will not get absorbed and the food will accumulate and contribute to heaviness. Practice visualizing your body comfortably receiving the food you eat and all its nutrients, so you can feel comforted, on all levels, and be comfortable indulging yourself in the pleasure that food can give.

Eating For A Happy Digestion

Digestion is at the heart of you feeling lighter, in both mind and body. Whether it be your microbiome, gut flora, stress related digestive issues or specific foods disrupting your digestion, this is something that you need to address and strengthen, and is a daily practice requiring your conscious awareness.

We will deal your digestion in detail later, but for now I would like you to begin incorporating these practical tips for a BeUtiful digestion at every mealtime starting today:

» Chew Your Food - Your wonderfully intelligent digestive process begins as you first lay your eyes on food. Without even taking a bite, your digestive juices are preparing to get to work on the food you're about to eat. Once the food is in your mouth, chewing is the next essential step in the digestive process, and if missed, has the potential to completely sabotage the rest of your food's journey through your body. Even more disturbing is the effect on your waist line, not chewing your food properly will add inches to your stomach as partially digested food accumulates creating gas, bloating, and excess water. Other side-effects are over-eating and feeling unsatisfied with food. Your brain takes about twenty minutes to register that you are full. If you are not chewing properly then you have likely inhaled your way through double what you needed, only to feel like you are about to pop later on. To taste food you need sufficient saliva. If the food is not in your mouth long enough to allow this secretion to properly stimulate the taste buds, the flavor and pleasure is completely unrealized. Chewing also alkalizes food, this is essential for a healthy acid-alkali balance and will also eliminate bloating and gas. If you are making the effort to eat nutritious healthy food, then you must chew your way through every last bit to get the nutritional benefit. How do you chew properly? The idea is that your food doesn't leave your mouth until it is liquid and its original form becomes unrecognizable. Remember, your stomach doesn't have teeth. Chewing your food around 30-40 times is suggested as optimal but you may need to build up to this. Meal times will take longer, but you will feel fuller quicker, eating less food but absorbing more nutrition.

» Don't Drink Whilst Eating - In Ayurveda, drinking a lot water whilst eating is like poison for the digestive system. The water dampens your digestive fire and dilutes the necessary digestive enzymes to break-down food. This means you are more likely to suffer from indigestion, bloating and a build up of undigested, toxin forming food in your stomach. If you have been really careful about what you eat but still feeling heavy and bloated after meals this could be the reason why. Ideally, drink water at room temperature 30 minutes before you eat and then not again until a 20-30 minutes after your meal. A few sips during your meal is fine, but try to avoid anything more than this. Even worse for your digestion is drinking fruit juices and sodas, so definitely avoid these at mealtimes. If you do feel heavy after eating, wait 30 minutes and then sip hot water, the heat of the water can help settle digestion.

» Don't Ignore Your Hunger - How often have you tried to ignore your stomach rumbling when you're on a diet? Those hunger pangs have been seen as the saboteur of your best weight-loss efforts but this is not the case. Ignoring your hunger is an absolute disaster for your digestion as it create excess gases, bloating and a slower metabolism. If you're feeling hungry your digestive fire is all geared up for food, but if you don't eat then this fire has nothing to burn and this creates an imbalance as your stomach literally 'turns on itself'. You must listen to your body, eat when your body is asking specifically for food, and try not to go any longer than four hours without eating.

» Bless Your Food - Take a moment before you eat, look at your food, appreciate it, thank it for nourishing your body. Your relationship with food, and foods relationship with you, starts the moment you start thinking about it. The more loving your intention before you eat, the more positive energy you are infusing into this relationship, and the easier your body will digest the food. Thoughts are energy, food is energy, use your energy of intention wisely. Calm yourself, breathe, and slow down enough to be conscious of the interaction that's happening the moment you sit down to eat. For a BeUtiful body this process, or ritual, of eating needs to be a BeUtiful one and filled with self-love, awareness and appreciation.

Self-Test Food Intolerances

Food intolerances, left undiagnosed, sabotage your digestion and ability to feel light, so we need to get to the root of these, if you have any, before we go any further.

Different to food allergies, intolerances are nothing to do with an immune system response, but rather are solely digestive related. Symptoms will vary according to the individual but can include bloating, weight-gain, difficulty losing weight, gas, IBS, headaches, sleepiness, anxiety and hyperactivity. This is why conscious and intuitive eating is so important, and why food journaling can highlight foods that maybe triggers to these unwanted symptoms.

There are many tests that you can do to find out about your suspected food intolerances, however, if you don't want to go this route of testing I have some practical advice that you can use daily, as this does not need to be over-complicated.

First of all, the 'problem' food is going to be something that you eat regularly, daily even. It isn't the food you eat once per month that causes you regular discomfort. Look through your daily diet and notice which foods are creeping into your mealtimes on the most frequent basis. These foods are the first to experiment with eliminating as over-eating of a specific food directly contributes to intolerances.

Wheat, meat, sugar and dairy are common culprits, but I have created food intolerances by eating oats every single day, and have done the same with vegetable juices. One of my clients said she had been eating salad, the exact same salad, every lunch and dinner time for the past year, and she wondered why despite this, her stomach was heavy, bloated, and uncomfortable. I suggested she stopped eating that salad! After her initial shock of no more salads she was worried that she'd put on weight. She had been strictly controlling her calorie intake for a year, with salad being one of the lowest calorie foods, she felt safe eating it.

After much assurance and persuasion, she gave it a go and ditched the salads for warmer soups, stews, roasted vegetables, and stir fries. The results were amazing, it was like someone had put a pin in her stomach and it had deflated. She could hardly believe it, the bloating had gone and she was feeling comfortable in her stomach. It is common to think that feeling uncomfortable after eating is normal, it isn't. If you are eating and feeling anything other that comfortable and satisfied, then something is wrong.

Ideally, if you notice a specific food causes you digestive issues, avoid it for three months, and then slowly begin to reintroduce it, if you feel you want to, and be conscious of your body's response.

You can also do the pendulum test, (Eden, 1999) to find out which foods will have a negative or positive effect on your system. I found this tool wonderful for building up a positive relationship with food as you experience your body 'wanting' a specific food and trying to get away from others.

To do the pendulum test for yourself follow these steps:

» As you are deciding what to eat, hold the food in your hands in front of you and draw it toward your stomach so that your arms are straight down your sides with your elbows bent at a 90 degree angle

» Stand up straight with your feet together and relax your body by breathing deeply

» Ask your body to show you if this food is helpful for your body right now

» Now take a deep breath in and exhale through your mouth, with a sigh of relief, and allow your body to move instinctively

» Notice if you move forwards, backwards or stay steady, the movement may be very subtle for some foods and more pronounced for others

The results - if your body moves forward, that is, toward the energy of the food in your hands, then this suggests it's a good food to eat right now and will have a positive effect. However, if your body moves backwards then it's trying to get away from the energy of the food. which suggests it wouldn't be the best choice for your body right now. If your body doesn't move in either direction then there is no strong reaction to the energy of the food and will be fine to eat, having no significant positive or negative effects on your system. This can change from day to day, so re-testing is a great way of building a more accurate picture of what works for you, and when, and what doesn't.

In many ways, this test is more sensitive than other testing methods as it is relative to the moment, how you're feeling, your energy levels, how strong you are today and how your digestion is for example.

This testing process really helped me to reduce my fear of food. It is so nice to feel your body move toward something that it wants to eat for the nourishment and the energy of a particular food. This is a powerful way to get connected with your body and begin a more inspired, body wisdom led approach to nutrition.

Taste Your Way to Feeling Lighter

As we are working on becoming more conscious and 'in tune' with what we eat and how, I want you to generate more awareness of how your food tastes. We are sensual beings, therefore the more we learn to engage more of our senses when it comes to food, the more holistic our approach to caring for our body will become. Relying less on text books and food arithmetic, and more on our senses and instinct, literally feeling our way through each and every food choice and mealtime.

Specifically, in Ayurveda, a model of traditional Indian medicine, there are six identified tastes that encompass all foods. They are:

1. Sweet

2. Sour

3. Salty

4. Bitter

5. Pungent

6. Astringent

Each of these tastes affect the body, or the elements in the body, in a different way. For example, sour tastes create more water. Imagine sucking on a slice of lemon, your mouth begins to water, this is one way sour increases the water element in your body.

All tastes have positive healing affects in moderation. However, your particular constitution, or dosha, will determine which tastes you should have more and less of. You can take a quick and easy online test if you go to Deepak Chopra's website and find out which dosha you are according to Ayurvedic principles. This can be really helpful in fine tuning your system to experience a more balanced state whilst reconnecting you with the elemental nature of food.

However, for feeling lighter there are three tastes that are identified as essential to counteract heaviness. They also happen to be the most under eaten of all the tastes – bitter, pungent and astringent.

If you are eating too many sweet, salty, and sour foods, relative to bitter, pungent and astringent, then you may struggle to create lightness in your body. Think about the taste of your food throughout the day, even if it's not sugary, it is easy to consume a lot of 'subtly sweet' foods like cereals, bread, rice, fruits and sweet tasting root vegetables. I don't want you to eliminate these foods, they're all excellent for soothing the body and reducing stress, but it is a good idea to be conscious of incorporating all the tastes, in a ratio that feels good for your body, relative to your constitution.

Here are the foods that within Ayurvedic principles cut through fat and heaviness, and promote lightness in your body. It is a good idea to incorporate a selection of these on a daily basis. For example, if I eat pasta, usually buckwheat pasta, or avocado on toast for example, I will always include a bitter leafy green like rocket or arugula, to counteract the sweet and oily nature of the pasta and avocado. This also helps me to better digest the food I eat, working with the elements to help my body breakdown what I'm eating so I can stay feeling comfortable and light. Take a look at these foods and see if you can bring a little more balance to your mealtimes and incorporate a wider range of tastes to encourage more lightness:

» Bitter: Detoxifies and lightens tissues – bitter greens, dark leafy greens, spinach, turmeric and fenugreek.

» Pungent: Stimulates digestion and metabolism – chili peppers, cayenne, onion, ginger, garlic and spices.

» Astringent: Absorbs water, tightens tissues, dries fats – legumes, pears, apples, broccoli, cabbage and cauliflower.

Part 3 - You and Your Body

*The relationship between you and your body defines
the energetic, and therefore, physical environment
within which all of your cells and bodily systems are
functioning. The environmental condition of your body
is what determines the health of your cells and how well
your bodily systems perform. Therefore, the difference
between loving and hating your body is ultimately the
difference between health and dis-ease, lightness and
heaviness in your physical experience.*

Body Talk

What is your body? Have you ever asked yourself this question?
I hadn't, the thought of what my body was had never entered my
head. I just felt my body was heavy and fat, so that's what it was, end
of conversation.

Get your BeUtiful Body journal and note down your feelings to this
question:

> » *What is my body?*

I ask my clients this question, at first they think it's silly and a waste of time, eyes rolling in the back of their head type thing. But as they slow down and consider this seemingly obvious question, they begin to understand the significance.

Your first answer may be something like, "well, my body is skin, bones, and flesh with organs that keep me alive." But is that it? Is your body merely a bag of bones bound by skin?

Let's put it this way, if your body is simply skin and bone, then why do you have such strong feelings about it? What's all the fuss really about?

Well, the fuss is because your body is a significant part of your self constructed identity. You look at your body as a direct reflection of who you are. This is why it feels so important to have a body that you like. You've pinned a significant part of your self-worth on how your body looks, and so too it seems, has the rest of the modern world. Understandably then, there is an ocean of emotion invested in how your body looks.

Conversely, from a 'spiritual' perspective the physical body is temporary and therefore, attaching any self-worth to it totally undermines all that you really are. I agree. But, hearing this doesn't help very much when you are in the midst of a body crisis feeling terrible.

However, by infusing your physical focus with this spiritual wisdom creates a way forward that provides relief from the type of body crisis that taints the lives of so many women. Becoming aware that you are more than just your physical body and that it is the most 'temporary' part of you, whilst from a place of self-love, creating a body that feels good to live in and that reflects the light and beauty that you naturally are.

Your body won't be here forever, fact, but your energy will be - according to the laws of physics, energy cannot be created or destroyed, only transformed. But your body is 'home' to U right now, it is the temple that houses your spirit on this earthly plane. So your body does matter, just not in the way you've been trained to believe since you were a little girl!

Your Relationship With Your Body

"Our biography becomes our biology."

Marianne Williamson

The type of relationship you have with your body is a daily choice of thought and action. Too often this relationship, instead of being based in appreciation for your body, is more heavily weighted toward not feeling good enough. The problem is, when you don't feel good enough this becomes your experience because you physically create what you think and feel. Your biography literally does become your biology, and not the other way around, and your relationship with your body is the channel through which all of this information is flowing.

This is an important distinction to make, too often all efforts to change or improve your body, or your biology, are purely physically based, like dieting and medicine, without any appreciation of the creative nature of your emotional state. Your life feels like it's 'on hold' until you get the body you want, but you never get the body you want because your relationship with your body is tainted with a poor body image and a huge lack of self-love.

Liberating yourself from what you think your body 'should' look like and loving it regardless, is the quickest way of encouraging your biology, and your dress size, to be exactly what you want - healthy and light. This is the complete opposite of what mainstream diet and beauty efforts have been teaching and as a result, we've been pushed into an unprecedented era of body crisis.

Body Crisis

Recall one of those mornings when you wake up and feel completely out of sorts, for no apparent reason you just feel heavy and irritated in your skin. In reality you look no different from what you did yesterday, and yesterday you were in your skinny jeans feeling fine.

As you're scanning your wardrobe, this heavy bloated feeling gathers momentum as you frustratingly flick through your clothes. You can't see anything that you want to wear, and you get that sinking feeling that nothing is going to look good on you today anyway.

You finally pick something and throw it on because now you're late. You hit the rush hour traffic, you look in the rear view mirror and you don't exactly shower yourself with compliments!

The rest of the day is spent feeling increasingly more uncomfortable as 'body crisis' gets into full swing. You either starve yourself for the whole day or do the total opposite and eat everything! By the time you get home, you're exhausted and irritated whichever which way your day went with food, too much or too little, neither work well for a light feeling body. The more days you have like this the further away you move from your BeUtiful body.

The real 'crisis' though is that we are passing this dysfunctional behaviour on to younger generations. Girls are dieting and having weight challenges at ages when it shouldn't even be in their vocabulary. A study by the US Department of Health reported that half of 9 - 10 year old girls are dieting and almost half of the children between 1st and 3rd grades "want to be thinner"[20]. Little girls are worrying about their body and forming negative body images, even before they've bought their first bra. We are, quite literally, feeding it to them and it needs to stop.

We need to stop being so judgmental of other women's bodies, and our own. We need to stop the shaming and hating of other women's bodies and of our own. It makes me cringe when I see glossy magazine 'before and after' pictures of celebrities who've apparently "exploded to a size 10!" I mean really, is this a civilized, let alone kind, way to be talking about each other? Collectively, we need to heal from all this body hating because the damage, pain and dis-ease being caused is detrimental to not just you, not just women, but to all human kind and Mother Earth. This isn't how we should be treating each other, and it isn't how we should be treating ourselves.

Can You Say... "I am Beautiful"?

The moment you embark on any self-healing journey, whether that be physical, emotional, or spiritual, there is one inescapable message. It doesn't matter which book you are reading, guru you are following, yoga you are practicing, meditation you are contemplating, retreat you are considering, or detox you are braving, this message weaves its way through all of it forming the foundation upon which the art of healing rests. The message is simple, the message is love, self-love.

As simple as it sounds, loving yourself doesn't always feel easy. Being kind to yourself can feel extremely challenging, and the idea of proclaiming that you think you're beautiful, well, completely out of the question! I mean, who does she think she's is?!

Innocent giggles aside, it does seem that a woman who has found a way of practicing self-love and admiration for her body is not always well received, "OMG, she just loves herself too much," is an all too familiar criticism.

I noticed this when I was a little girl. I never felt beautiful, far from it, so it wasn't a statement I was ever about to make, but I did witness the toe curling reaction of my friends to girls that did have a certain air of confidence about their appearance. I found this fascinating and I can remember thinking to myself, I don't understand, don't you all want to feel beautiful and confident like she does?

As teenagers this only gets worse, self-love is definitely out and self-deprecation is well and truly in!

Unfortunately, self-deprecation seems to stay 'in' and even as grown conscious women, self-love stays out! It feels jaw clenching for us to proclaim to the world that we are in love with ourselves and say "yes, I am beautiful." To admire a woman for her beauty is one thing but if she appears to acknowledge this herself then that's something entirely different and apparently not so pretty!

The question is, why? Why is it that when another woman is in love with herself and can say aloud she's beautiful, regardless of her dress size and appearance, instead of celebrating and supporting her, we want to judge and criticize?

We all want to feel love, and beauty is an expression of love. The truth is, when we are not feeling something that we really want it's irritating to be confronted with someone who does, and for all the judgement and criticism we give out we are giving it back to ourselves in even bigger doses.

As a teenager and young woman, I did not feel beautiful, quite the opposite, and for a very long time, hated my body and treated it badly. But, even throughout all of this, when I did see a woman, confident in her beauty and loving herself, I never contributed to the 'hating.' I always admired her, quietly thinking "wow, I'd love to feel like that." It was the feeling that I connected with most, not necessarily the physical appearance, I understood that beauty could not be measured, judged or compared!

Life is fascinating because this became my journey and my work, to find the beauty within me and learn to love myself so that I can help other women to see their beauty and feel their own love, too.

It's an amazing thought to consider how life would be if we all supported each other in loving ourselves, congratulating our sisters when they discover the beauty within them, and enjoying the pleasure of celebrating all of our unique, beautiful natures.

If we want something, we must learn to give it. Perhaps we could begin by giving our love and appreciation, instead of judgement and criticism, to all the women in our lives, including those who are already embracing their body's and feeling beautiful. In doing so, we create a window of opportunity to gift ourselves permission to love ourselves and reconnect to our beautiful nature.

Let's do something about this now. Rather than sitting around waiting for someone to tell you that you're beautiful, start telling yourself. Start telling other women, stop buying magazines that body shame other women, stop negatively gossiping about someone else's body, or your own.

"The thing women have yet to learn is nobody gives you power. You just take it."

Rosanne Barr

We already have the power to make a new choice that supports our collective wellbeing and reclaims the sovereignty of our own physical body, so let's use it! I want to get as many women as possible to make this BeUtiful promise, to themselves and to each other and I want you to make a promise to yourself right now. If you take this promise seriously, you will not only be helping womankind, but you will be creating an inner environment that is conducive to creating your most BeUtiful body as you embrace a more loving relationship with your body.

A BeUtiful Promise

I consciously choose to love and respect my body, looking only through kind eyes and practicing non-judgment. I speak only words of appreciation for my body and I share this love and respect for every other woman's body and honour our shared divine feminine beauty. I see the beauty within me and I see the beauty within you.

With Love......................

In Lak'ech A'la K'in. I am you, and you are me. Each time you judge another, you judge yourself. Each time you criticize another person's body, it hurts, them and you, because you can't criticize another and at the same time not criticize yourself. Those that judge others the most are often in the most pain from the judgement they inflict upon themselves! Make the BeUtiful Promise to yourself, and help others to do the same.

Conscious Loving

As soon as we look to food as a tool to help create the body we want, we become very conscious of the food we are putting into our body, each day, breakfast, lunch, and dinner. But how conscious are we about how much love we give our body? Are we consciously loving our body to the same degree that we are consciously feeding ourselves, are we practicing self-love morning, noon, and night?

Think about your most loving relationships, how do you show your love? Do you say "I love you", or maybe you share affection, kisses, and cuddles? You show your love in whatever special way that you do and, in a healthy relationship, all of this is returned to you. This 'sharing of love' feels blissful, connected and happy. In contrast, when love isn't shared and expressed, the relationship feels like the exact opposite, stressful, unconnected and unhappy.

If this is the case for your relationships with others, just imagine the case for the relationship with your own body. Your body needs your attention, it glows when it feels loved and appreciated, your cells come into balance with ease and you allow your natural state of wellbeing.

Conscious love, like conscious eating, has to be on the menu, daily, morning, noon and night, for your body to feel the benefits of your love and appreciation. You need to remind your body that it's safe, that you are caring for it, nourishing it, and have respect and appreciation for how intelligent and perfect it really is.

Not hating your body is not enough, stopping the insults and criticism isn't enough. Your body, needs your love, it needs conscious loving.

"You must love your body. And then lovingly give it food. And when you love your body and lovingly give it food, it matters not what food you give it." Abraham Hicks

Conversations With Your Body

What was your last conversation with your body? A typical conversation that I used to have went along the lines of, "why can't you just be thinner, what's wrong with you?!"

Take a moment to consider the conversations you're having with your body on a regular basis. Are they love filled? Or are they full of criticism? You can't change what you're not conscious of. Most of the conversations I used to have inside my head about my body were so frequent I didn't even know I was having them, it was automatic, habitual even, to have constant negative dialogue about my body.

To be able to change I had to first become aware of what I was thinking and telling myself. As I made an effort to notice what thoughts were going through my head I was so shocked at how many there was, daily, hourly, it was exhausting. But little by little, as I became more aware I was able to stop the negative thoughts and replace them with something more loving. This is a conscious choice I still have to make today, in line with my BeUtiful promise I made to myself.

Telling your body, morning, noon, and night that you love and appreciate it is the best medicine, there is nothing to rival the healing potential of your own self-love, and you couldn't get a more beautifying nutrient.

Shortly before her death, Mother Theresa said that loneliness and isolation in the West was the most significant 'disease' she had encountered during her lifetime, and indeed, scientific research supports her as studies have shown that love heals, whilst stress and negative thinking, including fear, can actually speed up the growth of cancerous cells and their spreading around the body[21].

The more connected we feel, to ourselves and to others, the more love we share, with ourselves and others, the more oxytocin gets released by the pituitary gland and heart. Interestingly, the more oxytocin in our system the less we crave drugs, alcohol and sweets!

Referred to as the "love hormone", oxytocin has also been called "the hug hormone, cuddle chemical, moral molecule, and the bliss hormone due to its effects on behaviour"[22] and how we feel.

Regardless of what your body looks like right now, the fact that your heart is beating, your lungs are breathing, and your mind is conscious, is a good enough reason to love your body. It has survived your lack of love, just think what would be possible if it actually received your love! This can happen right now, in this moment you could chose to love your body and it would instantly feel the benefit, and you'd know it because it would feel like relief.

"All you need is love."
John Lennon

Light Thoughts

Thinking 'light' thoughts about your body doesn't sound like the most effective diet plan, but research suggests that thinking negative thoughts about your body creates low self-esteem and an unhealthy relationship wth your body. When you have an unhealthy relationship with your body, or anything or anyone for that matter, your actions within that relationship tend not to be the healthiest, most love-filled choices that reap positive benefits.

Also, if you factor in the law of attraction, then you can't think one thing and expect something else to manifest. You can't think negative thoughts, thinking how heavy your body looks for example, and then expect it to feel lighter anytime soon.

Most often, the law of attraction is talked about in business, and that you have to 'think positive' and 'feel abundant' to attract money and generate success. However, the law of attraction, the law that says like attracts like, is hardly ever mentioned in the context of diets and weight. Yet the power of thought is so relevant for wellbeing and your physical experience because all healing starts in the mind.

If you are yet to fully appreciate the relevance of your thoughts in the conversation of your weight, then please allow me to be crystal clear. Your body's weight and state of health is a direct product of the thoughts you think, which are underpinned by your beliefs. Yes, food does matter, but your beliefs, thoughts and intentions about what you eat and your body are what create the inner environment within which food gets digested. A, so called, 'healthy' diet cannot override or erase the damage of stress, negativity and an unhealthy relationship with your body.

There are people eating all types of food, in a variety of different ways and in varying quantities, and the food equation cannot predict that those that eat the most weigh the most. Conversely, there are people eating very similar diets and yet experience completely different physical results. Something other than food is influencing your body.

Diets are a waste of effort when you're constantly thinking thoughts that are in direct opposition to what you are wanting to create. You have to streamline your thoughts and focus your mind, this will nurture a more positive and balanced emotional state, and then, with emotional stability, you have empowered yourself to be able to make the most inspired, conscious choices for you and your body.

Thoughts and emotions are energy, they are a creative force in their own right. Unfortunately, you sabotage your best eating efforts with thoughts filled with negativity about food and your body, and then you think your body is somehow against you. Your body isn't against you, your mind is, and you need to get your mind focused positively on what you want.

"When you feel fat your food makes you fatter - it does! When you feel slender your food keeps you slender - it does! You must understand that because you see people eating similarly with very different results, and you say, "oh yeah, it's their metabolism," and we say, "what do you think metabolism is?!" Metabolism is a vibrational response to your moment in time. Metabolism is the way energy is moving through your body, you see. And so "everything" is in response to the way you feel. Everything is. Everything is mind over matter."

Abraham Hicks

Stress - Damage Limitation

Stress is one of the major root causes of all health issues, essentially because it has a very real physical impact within your system, creating acidity and imbalances all over the place. Your digestion especially suffers, as under a state of stress all energy is diverted away from non-essential systems for your survival, so digestion practically gets shut down. Stress, therefore, is a major contributor to digestive issues, poor metabolism and heaviness.

High stress levels also cause adrenal gland fatigue. If you want to feel lighter you need your adrenal glands to be happy, believe me. Symptoms of adrenal gland fatigue include difficulty losing weight, cravings for sweet or salty foods, weak immune system, difficulty getting up in the morning, insomnia and mild depression.

Your adrenal glands are also closely related to your thyroid gland and this often suffers as a consequence of high stress levels too, meaning your metabolism is compromised even further. Adrenal gland fatigue isn't the only stress induced health challenge, but it directly impacts your ability to get your body to feel lighter, with typical dieting and exercising approaches tending to make it worse.

In addition, stress produces a chemical response in the body that creates an acidic environment. It also disturbs the entire endocrine system, raising cortisol levels, and other stress hormones, compromising both digestion and immunity. In an attempt to neutralize this acidity, your body will retain water and you will have a greater propensity to accumulate fat, especially on your stomach.

Stress has the potential to make you heavier without even a sniff of a chocolate cake, and if your stress is a response to negative thoughts about your body then you can forget feeling light! Yet standard diets don't do anything to alleviate the impact of this stress and in fact, they create more of it!

As you go through this book I will help you to refocus your thoughts positively and nurture a loving relationship with your body, in the meantime there are three practical ways that you can help get stress out of your body right now, and, if practiced on a daily basis, you can achieve a significant reduction in the stress hormones that are lingering in your body tissues. Incorporate them into your daily routine in a way that feels good for you:

REBOUNDING

Rebounding for 20 minutes per day has been shown to be incredibly effective for the lymphatic system, helping to pump fluids around your body whilst enhancing your body's ability to cleanse and detox, literally flushing the toxins and stress hormones that are carried around in your lymphatic fluid through your system. It is an excellent form of exercise too, stimulating each and every one of your cells and muscles in your body whilst reducing water retention and building good core strength and balance. NASA approves of this and so does Alisa Vitti who runs a blog called FLO Living. I love this resource and have been inspired by many of her tips, especially for hormone related challenges.

MASSAGE

Your issues are in your tissues, accordingly to yoga and many body-work modalities, so touch really can heal, physically and emotionally! Self-massage is an essential part of your self-care routine as it promotes the feeling of love and support. The massage itself stimulates the lymphatic system and helps the toxins to be flushed though your system, rather than building up and creating a toxic burden. This really helps to de-stress your body, chemically as well as emotionally. If you can, self-massage daily for five minutes, using a natural oil like coconut or sesame oil. You could also add essential oils as you feel inspired. If you really feel your lymphatic system is sluggish castor oil is supposed to work wonders, especially massaged around your stomach and lower abdomen.

ORGASM

Yes! Orgasm also helps to flush stress hormones out of the tissues so they can be processed and cleansed from your body, leaving you feeling calm and relaxed. Yoga, meditation and orgasm are apparently the beauty and fitness regime of the modern goddess these days, and the more I research this, the more I am convinced of the power of these practices. Everything you can do to calm down, release tension and flush the stress hormones out of your body will have tremendous beautifying and lightening benefits, not to mention enhanced health and vitality.

Self-care and self-love practices are the recipe for a BeUtiful Body because they help to heal your relationship with your body! Start to integrate these on a daily basis, as it feels good for you. If you can get the stress out of your body then it will respond much quicker to everything else that we do later to help you feel lighter.

Eating For Peace

You can bring more peace to your to your body, through food. Here are some foods that have the potential to help you to nurture a more balanced, peaceful state whilst helping your body to deal with the effects of stress, on all levels. Energy follows thought so when you eat these foods, consciously remind yourself of why you're eating them, intention is powerful.

Remember to be conscious of how your body responds to them and use this feedback to inspire your choices next time.

» *Brown Rice and Oats* – both are soothing to the digestive system which generally calms your entire system and has a peace inducing effect on your mood. Choose gluten free oats to optimize the positive impact on your digestion - happy tummy happy mind! They also support your nervous system, hormonal balance, energy metabolism and directly help your body to deal with stress. Eat them warm to experience their most 'comforting' effect.

» *Bananas and Avocados* – with a rich, grounding quality thanks to their texture, both bananas and avocados can 'rescue' the body from a state of stress. Studies have shown that a deficiency in potassium increases your susceptibility to feeling stressed, and bananas are full of it! Avocados have 14 different minerals, including potassium, making them an excellent choice for replenishing your minerals that get so depleted during stress helping you to physically cope better. Avocado's are also alkali forming in your body, this is extremely beneficial for counteracting the acidity produced during times of stress.

» *Berries* – all of them, although my personal favourites are wild blueberries, the resurrection food according to Medical Medium, and goji berries for their free radical neutralizing antioxidant ability. A perfect remedy for stress damage, with Vitamin C to boost your immunity and strengthen your system so you can more easily regain your balance.

» *Green foods* – Mother Natures harmonizing foods are green. They restore balance to blood sugar and hormones, remineralize your body and neutralize harmful acidity. Green foods, when digested well, have the ability to calm, soothe and *cool heated emotions. Be conscious of your digestion when you choose between raw or gently cooked, smoothies or juices, of the following foods; spirulina, chlorella, seaweeds, celery, spinach, kale, rocket, broccoli, asparagus and bok choy.*

» *Sunflower Seeds – full of B Vitamins that are essential for healthy stress management and supporting your body. They are also rich in Vitamin E which provides excellent antioxidant support to keep cells healthy and protect them from then long lasting effects of a stressful state. These are best soaked to increase digestibility and nutrient absorbability. You could add 1 tbsp to your overnight oats as you soak them in water or a nut milk, or you could add to almonds for homemade almond milk to easily get more sunflower seeds into your diet without trying too hard. Or snack on sunflower seeds with goji berries, but make sure you chew them really well.*

» *Almonds – rich in essential fatty acid's and magnesium, they are excellent support for the adrenal glands, whilst balancing blood sugar levels and helping to keep you feeling sustained for longer. Soak them for better digestion and absorbability of their nutrients. Homemade almond milk is also an excellent, digestion friendly way, of incorporating more almonds into your diet. Even better, warm this up in the evening and add 1 tbsp of raw cacao powder, 1/2 tsp of cinnamon, a pinch of pink salt and a 1 tsp of raw honey or maple syrup for a beautiful hot chocolate that soothes as much as it beautifies.*

» *Herbal Teas – nettle tea is abundant in magnesium which raises serotonin levels (good mood hormone) and neutralizes the acid from stress, whilst valerian tea before bedtime will help you to get a peaceful night sleep and tulsi tea boosts your stress fighting prowess.*

Fear Not!

Getting the stress out of your body is one thing, but cutting it off at the source is another! Fear causes stress, and I certainly experienced a lot of fear in my relationship with my body, which caused me a great deal of stress. At the root of my challenges with my body was fear. Fear of being fat, but more than this, what I had associated with it, or rather, my belief system equating it to being undesirable, unworthy and unlovable.

Grab your BeUtiful Body journal and note down your first responses to these questions:

> » *Is your relationship with your body fear or love based?*

> » *Are you fearful of fat or heaviness?*

> » *Are you fearful of your body?*

> » *Are you fearful of food?*

> » *Why? What do you believe is at the root of this fear?*

Fundamentally, everything boils down to one of two things, love or fear. It sounds simplistic, but the most profound things usually are. My relationship with my body and food is a good example, there was no love, but there was a lot of judgement, measuring, worrying, analyzing and criticizing, all fuelled by a fear of not being good enough.

To acknowledge fear doesn't give fear more power. Fear is like chains around your body, pulling tighter and tighter, and it weighs you down. There was a time when I would have tolerated the fear if it got me what I wanted. Meaning, I would have embraced the fear, and 'did it anyway', if it meant I got thin and the heavy feelings kept their distance. But fear didn't keep me 'safe' from feeling fat and thinking negative thoughts.

Fear wraps around your body, like a dress two sizes too small, creating so much tension, restriction, anxiety and a build-up of pressure, that it's only a matter of time until your body bursts out of these metaphorical chains and swings to the other extreme. Your fear then gets justified as panic sets in from feeling out of control of food and your body and you watch the number on the scales go up and up, regardless of what you eat!

When you feel like this self-care is not at the top of your to-do list. Instead you get tough on your body, with a big dose of judgement and whatever extreme diet is being talked about most.

Fear does not release its grip on you, you have to release your grip on fear.

After working on my relationship with food and my body for quite some time, becoming an intuitive eater, practicing more self-love and care, I found myself wondering, out of curiosity, what if I decided to fear no longer? What if my worst fear was not realized because I managed to relax enough and choose love for my body? What if I surrendered to fear and chose love instead, what would my body naturally do when left to its own devices?

As I had this conversation with myself the thought came to me that my body is a part of nature, and just like everything else in nature, when in harmony with its own nature and environment, it thrives, and it does so efficiently, this means there is no lack, nor is there excess, just efficient, balanced, harmonious thriving.

The more you study nature, and the more you study the human body, the more in awe you cannot help but become. What if we have tortured ourselves with fear and the need to be in control, and it was completely unnecessary? Meddling with what is already a perfectly formed, fine-tuned, beautiful human body that effortlessly remains at its optimum weight under conditions of self-love and acceptance?

Has the need and pressure for us all to conform to one definition of beauty, instead of embracing our own uniqueness, created such a distortion that we have simultaneously created vast extremes of eating disorders, starvation, and obesity, not to mention, hormonal imbalances and other health issues? And, in doing so, have we opened the door to an endless line of dis-orders and dis-eases?

It seems that meddling in our own nature has created such disharmony that we can't stand the feeling of our own body. We have taken the natural and made it completely unnatural, and the most troubling part is that fear has made it feel like it's unnatural to feel light.

So what is beyond fear? Beyond fear is love, in fact fear is like the closet underneath the stairs, dark and scary, but when you reach for the light switch the darkness disappears and light fills the space.

Love is powerful, so you don't have to focus on overcoming fear, all you have to do is choose love, in every moment, and it is a conscious choice, day by day. By choosing love, you are simultaneously choosing balance and lightness.

Conscious eating is important, but conscious loving is essential. Without consciously loving your body, conscious eating is of no use.

Part 4 - You and U

At the heart of your life experience is your relationship with U, or rather, how connected you are with your ultimate self, with love. This connection is the most powerful force in your creative potential, including the manifestation of your physical body, calling all of your cells, all pieces of yourself, to function in peaceful union, as One. The more you BeU, the more love that you feel, then the healthier you will Be and the brighter your light will shine.

Your Relationship With U

Your relationship with your Self is the most important and influential relationship from which all else springs. The state of this relationship influences your relationship with everything else, with life itself, including your body, food, your boyfriend, work colleagues and family. If there is a lack of love in your relationship with U, you can guarantee you will feel a lack of love everywhere else, the consequences of which will manifest, subtly or not so subtly, all over the place.

If you don't love yourself, then your inner dialogue will be full of negative thoughts and criticism about you, and every other relationship you have, including with your body and food, is under the weight of this negative self-talk. Drowning in this ocean of negativity, your self-esteem and confidence sink to new lows daily, as everyday feels like an exhausting struggle as you zap the life force right out of you. All of this is a consequence of disconnection from who-you-really-are, because if you were connected to All that U are, you could only ever Be in love with yourself.

In contrast, loving yourself nurtures positive, peaceful inner dialogue nurturing self-esteem and confidence, naturally. This spills over to love for your body and you easily feel at peace in your skin. In this state your self-love nourishes every aspect of your life experience, including your health, and your body naturally finds its balance and feels light merely as a consequence.

Talk about a chain reaction, from U to how light your body feels!

It's NOT Your Genes!

Whilst we can explain the connection between U and your health experience using energy and vibration, I keep bringing your attention back to this for good reason, as mainstream science also proves the relevance of your relationship with yourself in relation to your health experience. Bypassing the classical biological model, that your genes are the determining factor in the health you experience, it is now understood that what happens in your mind is at the heart of your health, not genetics, so it really is all about U!

In fact, according to Bruce H. Lipton, PhD, cellular biologist and international best-selling author of 'The Biology of Belief' "only 1 percent of illness is actually related to genes. 99 percent comes from lifestyle." This is explained in the new model of biological science called Epigenetic's, control above the genes. "This means that the mind and the environment control the genes. If you have a positive belief about something, you send information that supports that reality about that belief. And with a negative belief you can manifest a negative thing."

We can see evidence of this in the 'The Placebo Effect', which is now considered to be responsible for 33 - 66 percent of all medical healing! Meaning it isn't just medicine that is helping people, it's their belief in their doctor and medicine that is. "So the power of thought is the control of epigenetic's."

The research by Dr. Bruce Lipton is ground breaking, and its consequences are profound, literally bridging our scientific and spiritual understanding of the human body. This is need to know information because it changes everything, everything you thought you knew about taking care of your health, losing weight, discovering beauty, it's all wrong! And this is why so many of us have been going around in circles, not getting any closer to what we want, despite monumental efforts!

Consider this; inside your body are 50 trillion cells, and every day you are losing billions of them due to aging, damage, wear and tear. Your body has to make new cells otherwise you'd run out of them and die! Your body does create new cells, these are called stem cells, they can become anything from bone, muscle, skin, brain etc.

In his own words this is Bruce Lipton's research, "I would take one stem cell and put it in a petri dish by itself. And the cell divides itself every 10 hours." "At the end of the week, I have 50,000 cells in the Petri dish.

The important part is that all the cells came from the same parent, so therefore I have 50,000 genetically identical cells. That is called cloning. So I have all these embryonic cells in the petri dish and they live in the culture medium, which is the environment. When I grow cells in a tissue culture artificially, I construct the culture medium based on the blood. That means I will make it according to the composition of the blood from the animal that I get the cells from. So when I work with mouse cells for example, I try to make a culture medium that is the same composition as the blood of a mouse.

So I grew one cell in a petri dish. After a week I had 50,000 stem cells. They are all genetically the same. And then I split them into three different petri dishes and have genetically identical cells in each petri dish. But I change the chemicals in the culture medium in each of the dishes. So in each of the dishes is a slightly different chemistry than in the other one. What happens is that in one dish the cells form muscle. In a second dish the cells form bone and in the third dish the cells form fat cells.

Now what controls the fate of the cells? The environment! They are all genetically the same. So if I change the chemistry of the culture medium, I change the fate of the cells.

People are made out of 50 trillion cells. So in a humorous way, a human being is not a plastic petri dish, but a human being is a skin covered petri dish. Inside your body you have 50 trillion cells in a culture medium. The culture medium is called blood. If I change the chemistry of the blood, it's the same as changing the chemistry of the culture medium in a plastic dish. It doesn't make a difference for the cell if it's in a plastic or in a skin dish, the cell is controlled by the culture medium. In a plastic dish this is a synthetic culture medium and in the skin dish the blood is the culture medium.

So the chemistry of the blood controls the fate of the cells. Now what controls the chemistry of the blood? The brain is the chemist.

The brain releases hormones and growth factors and signal molecules into the body via the blood and those signals go through the body and affect the cells wherever they are in the body. So the brain is the catalyst. And what chemical should the brain put into the blood? The answer depends on what the mind is perceiving.

So imagine you are sitting with your eyes closed, and you open your eyes and you see your partner and you feel love. So once you opened up your eyes and recognized your partner, the brain releases hormones associated with love like dopamine which is pleasure, oxytocin which is bonding and usually also growth hormones. So when people are in love, the brain is releasing a cocktail of chemicals including growth hormones. And those chemicals are adding strong nutrients to the culture medium, because they cause the cells to grow very healthy. So when people are in love, they have so much health that they glow.

Now you are the same person and you sit there with your eyes closed, but this time when you open them you see something that scares you. So what does the brain release? You release stress hormones and inflammatory agents that affect the immune system.

So if I take the chemicals that come out of the brain in love and put them in a plastic petri dish, the cells grow beautifully. If I take the chemicals that come out of a brain or person in stress and put that in a culture medium, the cells stop growing.

What your mind perceives is always interpreted. And you release chemicals from the brain that match what you see. If you see something beautiful, you release chemicals that give you growth. But if you see something that is threatening, you release chemicals that give you protection. And they are two opposite extremes in terms of what happens to the body. Growth is open, protection is closed. You cannot be open and closed at the same time, so we are either in growth mode or protection mode, but we can't be in both.

When we live in a world that supports us and our mind sees it as a healthy, wonderful, happy place, the chemistry from the brain goes into the blood and enhances growth. An environment that's threatening or scary releases chemicals of fear into the blood and that causes the system to shut down and go into protection.

The genes have nothing to do with this, because we haven't even talked about the genes. The control over the cells depends really on what the mind is perceiving or the mind is interpreting. The genes control nothing. Now there is this huge belief system that genes "turn on" and genes "turn off" which is not true."

So, are you open or are you closed? Are you in a state of love and positively or fear and negativity? If you are still looking at your body and hating it then you're in the latter, if you are still jumping on the bathroom scales and not liking the number you see then you're in the latter, if you are still restricting what you eat through fear of food you're in the latter, if you are not loving yourself then you're in the latter, closed, closed to your own growth and wellbeing, to your own light and beauty.

The Beauty in Being U

As Bruce Lipton's research tells us, the more you are in a state of love and appreciation, your body becomes healthier, you experience a greater sense of balance, your immune system gets stronger and your hormones start to feel happier. All of this naturally creates the conditions necessary for your most BeUtiful, light feeling body, as each one of your cells are happily working together in union under these conditions.

The greatest factor directly influencing your ability to consistently Be in this state of love and appreciation is a love filled relationship with U.

The greatest saboteur to you being in this essential state of love and appreciation is a negative, unloving relationship with U.

Underpinning your relationship with yourself is your connection to U. If you are connected to U, fully conscious and aware of your source energy and who-you-really-are in the greatest sense, it would be impossible to feel anything but love and appreciation for yourself, and others. So, the more you BeU, the healthier you are, the lighter you feel, and the more BeUtiful you become.

Being U is becoming conscious of what feels 'good' and what doesn't, and then taking action from this place of self-love, because you care enough about U to never compromise yourself. It's relaxing into yourself rather than trying too hard. It's following your wisdom and intuition rather than what everyone else is doing or what society tells you should be doing. It's the difference between effort and allowing, motivation and inspiration, dieting and intuitive eating, because you know you are love and light already.

The Dis-Ease When You're Not Being U!

At the root of all dis-ease and unhappiness is lack of self-love, which is ultimately a lack of connection with U.

When you don't love yourself you make choices, about food, lifestyle, relationships and basically everything in your life, that are not aligned with your true self. These choices are unhealthy, relative to you as an individual, and create imbalance, which produces a variety of negative symptoms that get expressed emotionally and physically in a multitude of ways depending on your constitution and unique body type.

These symptoms are your body's warning signal that something isn't right and needs your attention. However, most often these symptoms get ignored and so your body has to shout louder, making these symptoms worsen and/or multiply, in a bid to get your attention. When they finally do get your attention, now you're thinking something is definitely 'wrong' with your body and you go to the doctor, you get a diagnosis, and your mind believes 'this' is the problem, when in reality, it is merely a symptom of a lack of self-love, which has led to choices that are not fully supportive of your truth and highest good.

This 'mis-understanding' only cements the dis-ease further into your experience, because now you believe this diagnosis is the problem. And so, it is.

The 'problem' is your disconnection from the awareness of who-you-really-are, your true nature and the nature of the Universe. The solution is when you reconnect fully with who-you-really-are, your nature and the nature of the Universe. When you BeU.

> **"You are the only problem you will ever have and you are the only solution."**
>
> *Bob Proctor*

Get your BeUtiful Body journal and write down the following question and then begin writing whatever you feel inspired to write:

» *Is your body trying to get your attention?*

» *What symptoms of dis-ease are you experiencing, and why?*

» *What do you feel your body wisdom is trying to tell you?*

» *What different choices could you make that are more aligned with your body wisdom?*

Give yourself time to have this conversation, it isn't a one-off, it is a daily checking in with your body, connecting with yourself, creating time and space to be heard, loved and appreciated. U are your medicine.

Part 5 - Weight - The Whole Truth

Light on Weight

Your body isn't man-made, it is a feat of genius, complex beyond what today's biology has yet to fully understand, and crafted over 200,000 years of evolution and adaptation for the modern human body as we know it, according to the Smithsonian Institute.

Your body is a part of the natural world and follows the same laws of the universe like everything else in the cosmos. It is an intelligent organism, designed efficiently to move its way through this environment, surviving and thriving. Therefore your body isn't just holding on to excessive weight just for the fun of it, this would be a 'glitch in the matrix', inefficient and a complete waste of vital energy.

There is a reason for everything that is within your physical body, there is a reason for the health you experience and there is a reason for the weight that your body is manifesting. Therefore, excess weight, and any health diagnosis for that matter, is merely a symptom of imbalance somewhere in your system, emotionally and physically, rather than a problem in and of itself.

Speaking exclusively about heaviness, an imbalance in your system, usually having an emotional root that contributes to a physical imbalance, distorts the flow of energy in your body and allows for stagnation. This stagnation leads to accumulation which turns into heaviness. In this sense, a lack of flow means your body can easily start to feel heavy, lack of flow in blood, fluids, foods, nutrients, oxygen and vital life force energy. Thoughts and emotions also have the potential to stagnate and accumulate, leaving you feeling heavy, if you don't 'digest' them properly too.

It is highly likely that areas of your body that tend to feel heaviest, or accumulate weight, are also prone to tension, tightness and lack of flexibility. This is why yoga is so powerful, it is working directly to dissolve these energy blockages, freeing your body of stagnation and creating more flow, physically and emotionally.

When you begin to see your body in this way, as a complex, highly intelligent, interconnected system, rather than something just acting randomly and holding on to weight for no good reason, you 'real eyes' how you can approach your health and weight in a more holistic and inspired way. Seeking to correct your imbalance and enhance the flow in your body, on all levels.

Remember, there is never anything wrong with your body. The only question you ever need to ask, with regard to weight and any health diagnosis, is - what is your body trying to tell you?

Emotional Weight

One of my most significant realizations happened when I was in Nepal, trekking with my dad and brother. On this particular day, we were walking down from a small mountain village called Muktinath, a place of spiritual significance for both Buddhists and Hindus. We'd visited a temple and spent time watching people run through freezing cold showers of mountain water to cleanse themselves before going into the temple to make their offerings.

It was a beautiful clear morning, deep blue skies and bright sunshine, with the white snowy peaks of the mountains creating the most incredible contrast. We were at around 3,800 meters altitude, high enough to feel the need to consciously take deeper breaths to get the oxygen your body needs. It was an easy walk that day, thankfully, most of it was downhill, which was a relief because the day before had been mostly steep up hill.

Food, and the lack of it up in those mountains, was a major topic of conversation most days. It was interesting because my dad commented on how he hadn't eaten that much (for breakfast we had been served this pretty feeble looking watery porridge) yet he wasn't hungry and had loads of energy. I agreed and commented how surprising that was given how active we were. This made me think about fasting, and how it works. After an initial period of uncomfortable hunger, usually for the first three days, you tend to lose your appetite. This means your body is taking full advantage of the rest from food and turning its attention, and energy, to processing any excess and accumulation, whilst healing, repairing and rejuvenating cells. Hunger naturally returns when this 'work' is complete, and that means it's time to 'break your fast'.

Our bodies store toxins in fat cells, and as we lose weight these toxins get released into our system to be processed by the detoxifying organs, like the liver. Fasting aims to encourage this kind of toxic release, although it takes much longer than just a few days on a fast to reduce your toxicity on any measurable level.

But, what if unresolved emotional issues were also stored in a similar way? After all, emotional baggage that is packed with negative emotion is toxic too, just like physical toxins. This helps to explain why fasting is also an emotional, as well as physical, experience, with many people feeling emotional, irritated, and even depressed during a fast or detox, seemingly in the midst of these toxins being released, processed and cleansed. Traditionally, fasting rituals were centered around spiritual practice, with the restriction of food merely being consequential, but today this is not the way most people approach a fast and so its real magic and meaning is rarely experienced.

Ancient models of medicine and healing appreciated that our body is not just holding physical toxins, but also emotional toxins, which contributes to dis-ease and heaviness that accumulates in our bodies. In the context of weight, this helps to explain why there has been so much struggle around weight loss, and why it often turns into a never ending battle.

Our bodies are carrying emotional toxicity from every negative thought, feeling, and life experience that we've ever had and not sufficiently processed and healed. When we diet, sometimes we don't lose any weight, and other times we lose weight initially only to put it back on again the following week, month or year. Could this be because the emotional toxicity is still there and continues to weigh us down because we're not dealing with the root of the problem?

Like attracts like, and this emotional toxicity weighs you down, and overtime just attracts the physical manifestation of this same energy like a magnet. Over and over again, the weight physically gets attracted back on to your body, or never even manages to leave. This cycle, this yo-yo diet effect, will continue until you increase your awareness and finally manage to 'let go' of the emotional toxicity, all of those heavy thoughts, thinking you're not good enough, criticizing, judging, and comparing your body. I mean, forget the chocolate biscuits, this is where you need to lighten your load!

For me, my fear of being overweight was a huge part of my 'emotional toxicity'. Ironically, at my slimmest the fear was even worse. I'd also had the experience of my weight going up and then down without changing food or exercise, so I was already suspicious of something else, other than food, having a direct impact on my physical weight, or at least how heavy I felt!

This fear and my constant negative body image was emotionally toxic and was burdening my body. Even when I did manage to 'get' lighter, the fear and negativity was still there. Fear and negativity are energy, they have a vibration, and it was never that long until this vibration manifested itself physically and my weight would go up again. This vibration, or blueprint of my body, was still carrying the 'weight' of my toxic thoughts and emotions about my body, I had struggled, yet temporarily managed, to lose the physical weight, but, I was never able to lose the emotional weight, because, firstly I wasn't conscious of its power and so secondly, I wasn't trying to deal with it.

Remember I said my fear of putting on weight was always strongest when I was at my slimmest. Energetically, I was putting weight straight back on, rebuilding this information back into my cells every time I felt the fear of getting fat and thought negative thoughts about my body. My body had no choice but to recreate the exact image in my minds eye that all my fearing and negative body image had created.

"Your thoughts make you fat or thin, not your food."

Abraham Hicks

Open your BeUtiful Body journal and begin to write down your thoughts and feelings around these questions:

» *Are you fearful about eating?*

» *Are you fearful about your body weight?*

» *Are you fearful in life?*

» *Can you feel emotional toxicity within your mind or body?*

» *What 'baggage' are you carrying and would like to let go of?*

You can't change what you're not conscious of, this dialogue with your body is essential for the vibrational cleansing you need to create your most BeUtiful Body, easily!

Getting real about your 'emotional toxicity' is powerful, we will do loads more on this later, but for now, whenever you get into that place of fear or body shaming, practice this BeUtiful Imagination exercise to cleanse your mind and body of emotional toxicity. Remember, nothing will work unless you do, so you have to be willing to apply yourself to these practices, even though all you want to do is meddle with your food and 'gym' your body into whatever you want it to look like, because what's imagining going to achieve?! But, creating happens in your mind first, so this is where we have to start.

BeUtiful Imagination Practice - Allow your body to breathe, deeply. Slow your breath down, breathing in deeply and out completely.

Imagine what it would feel like to Be free from your own judgement and criticism. Imagine what it would feel like to think loving thoughts about your body. How much more ease you would feel as the stress of not liking your body begins to fade away?

Now, close your eyes and take a few moments to really imagine letting all of your negative thoughts about your body go. See those thoughts getting smaller and smaller, or hear those negative thoughts getting quieter and quieter, until you don't hear or see them anymore.

Just stay here for five minutes, breathing deeply, consciously relaxing your body and imagining yourself feeling light and beautiful. Enjoy this feeling.

The Secret Is Out

Being 'thin' is the Holy Grail of beauty, if you believe the propaganda of course. However, thin is not synonymous with beauty, but there was a time when I believed this was the case and it caused me a great amount of dis-ease! Do you believe that to be beautiful you have to get thin? Whatever that means these days because you can be too thin to be beautiful too, if you believe everything you read, so you just can't win if you play that game.

Ironically, whenever I did 'get thin', according to the scales, I definitely did not feel light! I feel lighter now, than I did when I was a dress size smaller. Working with so many women, I quickly realized this was true for them too, getting 'thin' and feeling 'light' isn't the same thing, even though reasonable logic assumes they would be.

During a consultation with a client diagnosed with anorexia, as thin as she obviously was, dangerously thin and close to hospitalization, she did not feel 'light' on any level, in her body, mind, or soul. She felt as heavy as lead, and what she saw when she looked in the mirror was a physical body that, despite being skeletal, looked exactly like she felt. How could someone so painfully thin not feel as light as a feather?

This got me thinking, what if our entire approach to diets has been fuelled by chasing 'a look' of thinness, because we've been told this is what would make us beautiful, when what we are really wanting is to feel light?

Ask yourself right now, what do you really want? Is it a look, or is it a feeling? Or is it both, and if it is, which comes first?

Are you chasing getting thin for the sake of the dress size, or are you seeking the feeling you believe the dress size will give you? At the heart of it, are you no just wanting to feel light? And, why would you want to feel light? Because, when you feel light you feel energized, when you feel energized you feel positive, when you feel positive you feel confident and when you feel confident everything is possible! So, isn't it true that what you are really wanting is a sense of freedom and liberation, to feel energy flowing through you so fast that you just feel so alive, inspired and full of light?

I said earlier that asking the right question was essential to make meaningful progress. Yes, you may want a certain dress size, but, only because you believe that in getting into that size, or seeing that number on the scale, you will feel better. Truth is that's not how it works because you're chasing an artificial 'look' rather than the 'real deal'. Why? Because weight loss and beauty are a business, and a dress size and a 'look' is what you're sold because it's a much easier sell than the 'real deal' of feeling light and being connected to who-you-really-are. The best part of the business model is that everyone's forever chasing because what they're chasing isn't real, it's manufactured, leaving everyone who is chasing feeling like they will never be good enough.

This directly impacts self confidence, and as a collective, drastically reduces the confidence of women. In numerous studies, the confidence gap has been identified as one of the leading causes of why men out-perform women in the workplace with higher pays and greater probability of promotion. Not because of ability or competency, but due to a lack of confidence within women, being more likely to be less self-assured than men.

The diet and beauty industry, whilst being cloaked in female empowerment, is one of the biggest contributors to female disempowerment of modern times.

If you want to feel light, if you want to reclaim sovereignty over your beautiful body, then break through your limiting, media imposed, notions of beauty and fixation on getting thin, and realize that in fact, when you seek your own light, when you connect with your true self, you connect with a power that has the potential to transform not just your body, but the world as you know it.

Get In Your Flow

Getting in your flow, on a mental level, naturally gives you confidence, as you tap into your inner knowing and genius. On a physical level, you also need to get in your flow to more easily connect with your body wisdom and begin to feel lighter.

However, when you're in the midst of body shaming and feeling heavy you get out of your flow and feel stuck, like nothing is moving and your body stubbornly holds on to every last inch, which gets you feeling all frustrated, exacerbating diet dramas and poor body image. However, this sense of being 'stuck' is only a perception, and it isn't accurate, because change is the only constant!

Your body tissues are in a constant state of recycling, as your cells are continually dying and renewing.[23] The cells on the inside of your stomach last around 5 days, the cells on your skin renew themselves every two weeks and your liver recycles itself once every twelve to eighteen months. Your body is in a constant state of renewal.

Becoming aware of this inner 'movement' and flow is powerful because instead of feeling stuck, allowing for stagnation, accumulation and heaviness to manifest, you understand that in every moment there are changes occurring in your body and you have an opportunity to create something you desire. Remember, your thoughts are energy, what you think you create and what you believe you see!

Being focused on 'feeling lighter' rather than 'getting thinner', more easily get's you in your flow. There is a 'river of light' flowing inside your body, carrying information throughout your entire system, from your thoughts and emotions to oxygen, blood, vitamins, minerals and food. The nature of life is constant flow, like the ocean's tides and currents flowing around the Earth, your body also has a natural flow that helps maintain its balance, harmony, wellbeing and lightness.

According to traditional medicine, emotions flow too as they are of the water element. Even though they can feel stuck and heavy at times, the more we understand the flowing nature of our emotions, of our body and of life itself, the more we are able to get in our flow and feel lighter, on all levels. Nothing is static, nothing is fixed, nothing is concrete or stuck, there literally is the opportunity for lightness in every moment, if we tune into our flow.

Nothing Flows Without Water

Water is fundamental to existence, without water there is no life!

Your energy and bodily fluids all naturally flow and it is from flow that your wellbeing and lightness springs, literally, because nothing moves without water!

Water is a brilliant conductor of electricity and energy, and since we are 'energetic beings' and our cells communicate by electric waves, then staying hydrated is vital for mental clarity, emotional balance and maintaining a high vibration.

Your brain is eighty-five percent water and dehydration has been noted as a contributing factor to senility, so a lack of water directly impacts your brains ability to function, as well as the nature of your thoughts. Basically, your brain becomes less functional if you do not have enough water in your system.

Water aids the cleansing process throughout your entire system, and all of detoxification organs love water too. Good hydration creates a clear body and mind. Water is also essential for optimal digestion, encouraging flow in your bowels too, which if you want to feel light is a very good idea. But how much water is enough? There is no one-size answer that will suit everybody, of course not. So again, it comes down to you being present and aware of your body to find the perfect amount relative to you. Obviously, this will change depending on how active you are, how well you slept last night, how much you've eaten, what you've eaten and your stress levels.

As a rough guide, two to three liters per day is a good amount to aim for, but this is not going to be right for everyone. If you struggle with headaches, lethargy, drowsiness, and have trouble concentrating, then you're probably not drinking enough water! Dry skin, dull skin and dark areas around your eyes also suggest you need more water. The color of your urine is an excellent indicator if all else fails. Ideally, the more pale in shade the more hydrated you are! Becoming more conscious of your body will help you to notice when you are thirsty. It is amazing how often you miss even the most basic requirements of your body when you're busy getting through the day.

When it comes to deciding which water to drink there is enormous debate, and in my experience all options have their pro's and con's. In an ideal world, we would be drinking fresh, natural spring water, straight from the source, unpolluted and without even coming close to a plastic bottle. Start from this premise and work your way to the best scenario for you, given your geographic location and water options.

To add to the water debate, a Japanese scientist named, Emoto Masaru, researched water and water crystals with fascinating results. He found that depending on the type of atmosphere water had been subjected to, it affected how perfect the crystals the water would create when frozen. He played classical music to one sample of water and heavy rock music to another. He said beautiful words like, 'I love you' to one and then 'I hate you' to another water sample. The more positive the 'input' the more perfect the water crystals, but when the 'input' was negative or harsh, the water crystals that were formed were distorted and mis-shaped.

These results are further proof that we live in a vibrationally based universe, and water, like everything else, including food and our body, is energy, reacting and responding primarily on an energetic level before manifesting into the more subtle layers, and finally resulting in the physical form.

Think of cells in your body like the water crystals. The more loving your 'inputs' into your inner environment, like your thoughts, emotions and food, the more 'harmoniously' your cells perform, creating a healthy, beautiful and light feeling body. However, if your 'inputs' are harmful and negative, full of toxins, both physical and emotional, then your cells will struggle within this harsh environment and are more likely to become 'rogue', essentially going against the greater good of the whole, creating a body of imbalance and dis-ease.

Morning Water Ritual

First of all, after I read that research I started putting my water on a piece of paper with 'love' written on it. Oh yes! Did I feel a difference? Well it did make me more conscious of love!

Whilst you sleep, your body is busy cleansing and restoring your entire system with attention paid to each of your organs, so you wake-up in the morning with a clean slate. To work with your body and enhance this process, the first thing that you need to put into your body should be hydrating and cleansing. Water. Not coffee!

This enhances your body's cleansing process, and prepares your digestion for breakfast. Avoid cold and iced water. This is a shock and induces stress, also, cold water isn't as hydrating as room temperature water. Drinking a large amount of water, for example, one liter before breakfast, increases bowel movements. If you change nothing else but do this, you will feel lighter!

Incorporating a Water Ritual into your morning routine is an excellent way to hydrate your body and infuse your internal environment with more love! Choose one of the following, or make up your own, and sip slowly and mindfully:

» *Warm Water – simple, cleansing and hydrating. This is a staple, if all else fails and time is short!*

» *Water & Lemon – using 1/2 a freshly squeezed lemon, this is cleansing, detoxifying and alkalizing.*

» *Water & Raw Apple Cider Vinegar - adding 1 tbsp of ACV to warm water, with a little raw honey if you need to sweeten. This ritual is antibacterial, immune boosting and detoxifying whilst also help-ing to boost digestion and promote proper pH levels in your body.*

» *Water, MSM & Vitamin C - not for the faint hearted, but one of the most powerful detoxifying things you can do to support and cleanse your system. It is also excellent for plumping up your skin, which makes the taste worth persevering with, and it increases hair growth! Begin with 1 tsp of MSM crystals and 1/2 tsp of vitamin C powder, stir well and drink. You can build up to 1 tbsp of MSM but keep the same dose of vitamin C. MSM (methylsulfonylmethane) is an organic sulfur containing compound that is used to lower inflammation, reduce joint pain, improve your immune function, encourage proper digestion, increase energy, reduce the effects of stress and many more health issues. Make sure you get a brand that is 100% pure MSM. It is powerful, so start at a low dose and listen to your body, especially your stomach, as it can cause diarrhea.*

» *Water & Milk Thistle Tincture - a natural herb used for over 2000 years. Milk Thistle is an excellent tonic for your liver which helps to strengthen its detoxifying abilities. It also supports digestion whilst being a great antioxidant. The tincture, liquid form, is the easiest for your body to absorb. Just add drops to water, as instructed on the label, and drink.*

Be Soft Like Water

Talking about flow and water invariably implies softness, as you can't flow without an element of softness. Perhaps this is why we have struggled to go with our own flow, not trusting our body wisdom, and instead wanting to follow external regimes and diets that gave the illusion of security. It is almost as if women's natural softness and changeable nature has been eroded by a rigidity born from external conditionality of 'body perfection'.

Someone once said to me that I'd gotten 'softer', I can remember feeling completely mortified, they might as well have said I was obese! It was actually meant as a compliment, it just shows how our insecurity can distort how we view things. Women do have 'softer' bodies than men, generally speaking, as women carry more fat than men do. But have we started to perceive this 'softness', physically and emotionally, as a hinderance rather than an asset? Are we trying to erase the differences in our biology along with erasing the inequality in the workplace, misguided under the illusion that 'different' automatically implies better or worse? Has the feminist movement tipped women toward emulating masculine energy, rather than celebrating the beautiful qualities of both the divine masculine and the divine feminine, each in their own right?

The feminine is soft but don't confuse this with weakness. Feminine is in constant motion, undulating, and fluid as our body dances to its monthly rhythm, expanding and contracting, feeling expressive and then feeling the need to retreat inward, this is the limitless nature of the female body and it isn't static.

The female body changes, just like the moon waxing and waning, the only constant is change, it will expand and it will contract. What is essential to know as a woman is, the less we try to fight and control this natural fluidity, the more in balance we will be and the less of the extremes we will experience as our body begins to fluctuate within a much smaller, more comfortable range.

When you stop fighting your body, it will stop fighting you. When you accept and embrace yourself, unconditionally, the fluctuations will be more subtle, the bloating and de-bloating less extreme, and with a greater sense of balance you more easily connect to your light and get into your flow, allowing your body to just Be.

> *"Become more feminine, more soft and delicate. Your ego is trying to create trouble. Your ego is saying to you, "Be strong, be masculine, be this and that." Don't go on that male chauvinistic trip - forget about it. Relax. Whatsoever is coming naturally is beautiful. This femininity has to be absorbed. It is not weakness; it is delicateness. It is softness that you are thinking to be weakness. To use the word "weakness" is to evaluate it. Your ego is evaluating it, condemning it - that this is something wrong, you are becoming weak. Ego always thinks of softness as weakness. That's why women down the ages have been thought to be the weaker sex. It is not true; it is false. Drop that word "weakness" - simply call it softness, femininity, and allow it. It is beautiful!"*

> *Osho*

To feel lighter make peace with your softness, and embrace it.

Body Wisdom Nutrition

Looking at your body as an intelligent, complex, interconnected system, you can begin to unravel the root causes of imbalance and heaviness, and how all of this interlinks with your vibration and emotions. The beauty is then, you can actually work with your body in an enlightened way, to feel lighter, naturally, and create your most BeUtiful body. All of this information has been life changing for me, because I finally started to understand my body, and understand myself, and with this came a sense of peace that I had never before been able to touch.

Spleen Energy - Nourish & Nurture

The spleen is a key organ that is very important in the management of weight. To intelligently address weight and create lightness, the spleen needs attention, failure to do so will certainly keep the weight roller coaster at full speed, not to mention disrupting digestion.

Your spleen is an organ that is part of the lymphatic system and it performs a wide variety of functions, including acting as a reservoir for blood which your body will call upon in an emergency. It is a major organ of filtration and is involved in the removal of old defective blood cells and the creation of antibodies and immune cells.

In Chinese Medicine, the spleen is considered an organ of transformation and nourishment. The spleen is also seen as holding a central point within the body and wellbeing depends on it, if the well runs dry then health and vitality are negatively impacted. For this reason, Chinese medicine will always look to strengthen the spleen and its energy, included its paired organ, the stomach, before addressing any illness.

For our purposes here, this is a key point. The spleen is also a primary organ of digestion, absorbing nutrients from food. If the spleen is not functioning properly then you're not able to absorb nourishment from food, or supplements for that matter, the nutrients remain undigested within the food and your body goes hungry. A strong spleen ensures that you are well nourished.

On a more subtle level, the spleen behaves in the same way with the idea of emotional nourishment. A weak spleen would mean that there would be difficulty absorbing emotional nourishment too, so when someone tell's you they love you, you'll find it hard to believe and take on board, starving yourself of that emotional nourishment.

Now this is really interesting, especially when we understand the link between being able to digest food and emotions well, and weight. When emotions are not digested it is more difficult for food to be digested too, and the combined effect is a toxic build-up of both. These emotional characteristics are one of the main precursors for challenges with weight, if you can't digest emotions well, and you can't digest your food then you will feel heavy.

If the spleen is weak then the body feels starved, it not only feels starved physically but emotionally too. In this state your body wants more, and you are compelled to give it more. As time goes by, how you fill this 'hole of neediness' becomes increasingly unhealthy. As the feeling of needing more keeps on growing, you seek out quicker 'fixes', physically and emotionally, but no amount of food seems to fill it.

The spleen also houses your inner 'mothering instinct', which as you get older becomes more prominent since you take over care duties from your mum as you become an adult. If spleen energy is not strong then this instinct to care for yourself is not as active as it should be. Instead of choosing food, lifestyles, friends, jobs, and exercise because they are beneficial, you find it harder to instinctively make choices that serve your highest good.

Mentally, the spleen is associated with the power of thought. The digestive process is mirrored on a mental level by the thinking process. You feel hungry, you eat, you digest and absorb the nutrients, or information, that your body needs. The same is true for knowledge. You want to know something, you get on Google, you read through, digesting and absorbing the information you want and forgetting the rest. Common phrases like "food for thought," "unable to digest the information," "verbal diarrhea," "eating my words," "chewing over an idea," all demonstrate this link.

There are more physical connections too, not being able to concentrate at work after eating too much at lunch time, losing your appetite when something terrible has happened or feeling as if you need comfort from food when you feel emotional or lonely.

How interesting that one of the primary organs responsible for receiving physical nourishment from food, is also connected with receiving emotional and mental nourishment. No wonder eating is such an emotional as well as physical process.

Emotionally, the spleen is concerned with feelings of care for both yourself and others. "A healthy concern for our own needs leads us to nourish ourselves emotionally and, if we are ourselves emotionally nourished, we can give appropriate nourishment to those we care about."[24] A healthy concern for our own needs is a pre requisite for being able to make positive choices, to nourish our body, mind, and soul. A lack of this 'concern' and appreciation is indeed the underlying factor of negative body images and harmful dieting.

Physically, a lack of spleen energy would indicate decreased digestive power and an inability to effectively absorb nutrients from food. The latter would certainly create a situation where you felt the need to eat more than you really need since you're not getting sufficient nutrition.

Emotional needs would also be left unsatisfied with weak spleen energy, also leaving you hungry emotionally as well and physically. This is a powerful combination when in the context of eating and lightness, if you are dieting and finding it difficult to feel lighter, miserable about your body, and feeling emotional then you need to strengthen your spleen energy.

On a more physical note, poor digestion is a huge culprit for gaining weight and difficulty losing it. A flat stomach is impossible with digestive issues, compounding the problem and adding more negative feelings and discomfort within your own skin.

When spleen energy is strong, Traditional Chinese Medicine says that you are comfortable within yourself, digestion is relaxed, you feel connected, able to nurture yourself and have a positive, almost motherly, relationship with yourself. Physically a strong spleen leaves the body supported, flesh is toned and firm, your mind is clear and you feel relaxed.

Understanding this, how can we continue to address weight without strong spleen energy? We can't, so we will be dedicating an entire week to learning how to heal and energize your spleen energy during 8 Weeks of creating your most BeUtiful Body.

Digestive Fire - Transformation

In traditional Chinese medicine, the spleen is paired with the stomach and this is where our transformational fire of digestion is found. A good strong digestive fire is essential to effectively digest what is consumed, on all levels, and this really is the driving force in your transformation. Fire is the ultimate transformational element.

You know all those people who eat everything and stay super slim, this is part of their secret. Strong digestive fires. When your fire is burning brightly, you eat food and it gets burned instead of stored, it's as simple as that. If your internal flame is waning, the food you eat is simply going to stay and grow heavy. When this happens, not only do you get that uncomfortable heavy feeling and struggle to get your weight down, but this food accumulation creates toxins, and these toxins cause bloating, gas, and other uncomfortable sensations.

Hormones, energy, skin, liver, heart, blood and lymphatic flow, everything is negatively affected if your digestion is weak. If you have this situation going on, it doesn't matter if your diet is 100% organic and super healthy, you won't be feeling energized and light at all, because the undigested food will be creating toxicity that will make you feel tired, bloated and heavy.

Digestive fire is fundamental to your health and wellbeing, on all levels, as not only do you digest food, you digest thoughts and emotions too. Therefore, a lack of digestive energy means that food, thoughts and emotions can get 'stuck' and stagnate, and then turn into toxic energy. Letting go of this toxicity is difficult without your inner fire of transformation burning up all this heaviness. Instead it lingers, weighs you down, and accumulates.

Epicurus was the ancient Greek philosopher was so enamored with the power and meaning of your digestion that he attributed good digestion to be the basis of all human goodness and that poor digestion was not only a precursor for poor physical health but also was morally destructive.

Your digestive fire is your power of transformation, this internal heat is what transforms food into positive energy to fuel your body, whilst burning up all the negative energy from toxic foods, thoughts and emotions. This internal flow of your digestive system is essential for you to feel light and positive. So we really can go as far as to say that any attempt to positively affect your health, wellbeing and weight, is incomplete if it doesn't address the strength of your internal fire.

Too much fire is obviously not good either, burning through your food too quickly can lead to malnourishment leaving you weak and feeling out of balance. As with everything, it is a fine balance that is needed, and the only way to find this is to become more conscious and aware of your own, unique, body.

After energizing your spleen to be able to take in goodness on all levels, we must enhance your ability to process it and turn it into positive fuel, your fuel for transformation! We will be working with this specifically during our 8 weeks too.

Liver Energy - Letting Go

Your liver is an absolutely amazing organ that is involved in a impressive volume of tasks within your body. A good strong liver is essential for you to be healthy, it is so important that it is the only organ that is capable of regeneration. This is an amazing feat that is not to be underestimated.

The liver is the major organ of detoxification. Everything that you eat and breathe gets sent to your liver from your intestines and your heart, and then travels through it to be cleansed, then clean, energized blood gets supplied back to the heart to be pumped around your body.

Remember how we said your spleen extracts the nourishment required by your body, and your internal fire is what burns through that and uses it for energy? Now think about the function of your liver. It is what gets rid of the rubbish after the fire, the liver is cleansing and eliminating all the stuff that your body doesn't want, usually, everything that's toxic!

Your spleen helps the body to absorb nourishment and the liver helps the body to eliminate waste. What a beautifully balanced system we have.

Crucially, your liver is also an important factor in the process of fat metabolism- breaking down fat to be used as energy. Your liver energy needs to be strong, therefore, to break down fat and process it as well as possible, dealing with all the physical and emotional toxicity within this process.

Your liver is associated with the emotions of anger, irritation, and frustration. We need to strengthen your liver to actively let go and 'detox' yourself from these kinds of energy vibrations. Doing so will allow for a smoother flow of energy around your body that is more comfortable and actively facilitating a lighter body as you let go of what no longer serves U, on all levels.

If you are 'dieting' without paying any attention to supporting your spleen, digestive fire, and liver then this will be a struggle. Since you can't release the toxicity that has contributed to your current state, your body isn't equipped to support it so the weight stays put, you feel miserable and frustrated.

When you crash diet, you may lose a few pounds or even meet your target weight, but the same inner environment remains, and it's toxic. It's also your point of attraction, since all of those toxins remain, along with all the 'thinking' that went into creating them in the first place! Right now we are detox crazy, going to all lengths to try and 'juice' the toxins out of our body, without even considering the toxins in our thinking, in our mind, or even strengthening the very organ that allows for detoxification in the first place. Don't waste your time juice fasting unless your liver energy is strong, you may lose a few pounds, only to be put on again when you start eating normally, but the real healing power of juice fasting is lost if you don't pay attention and nurture your livers energy and function.

Heart Energy - Unconditional Love & Light

Your heart pumps not just blood, but also life force throughout your entire system making the heart the ruler of your body whilst acting as a transition point between the physical and non-physical realms, in energetic terms. It governs emotions of love, harmony, balance, and acceptance, but your heart can be burdened with negative emotions like depression, guilt and can be exhausted through stress and worry. In this respect, it is really important that you learn to unburden your hearts with 'heavy' emotions that you've accumulated. Too often emotions overwhelm your hearts and they get suppressed, down to the lower regions of your stomach, leaving a black hole of emotional debris that feels too hard to deal with, and the flow of energy throughout your body suffers.

Sometimes, it's not even all 'your own stuff' that you find yourself trying to deal with. You have a tendency to be like sponges sometimes, picking up on things that are going on around you. If others are sad, you take on their sadness, if your partner is stressed, you feel their stress and worry. You are sensitive to the energy around you and if you don't take care of your own energy space then you pick all of it up, and most of it you can do without!

Taking on everything around us, the good and the bad, burdens our heart and overwhelms our entire system, making it heavy on all levels, especially if we can't digest and let it go efficiently. By managing our space in a more conscious way we are practicing powerful self-care. We are obsessed about calories in and calories out, but what about energy and emotions? If we were to pay as much attention to emotional energy that we consume as we do calories, we would all be a lot happier and lighter!

Being a 'sensitive kind of gal' has the potential to be fantastic if you realize it, and then learn how to deal with it in a positive way. But so often you're unaware, feeling crappy but not really knowing why. It's easy to think there's something wrong with you, you begin eating emotionally, feeling increasingly weighed down with no love for your body, your spleen suffers and you can't take in nourishment and feeling overwhelmed you're not able to filter out the rubbish either!

This is taking detox to whole new level, and goodness knows we need it! Cleansing our body, mind and soul, through food and thought, ritual and awareness, is essential.

Lightening the load stored in your heart will allow more light to flow through your body and this means you will be feeling the love, more and more, paving the way for self-acceptance, self-appreciation and self-LOVE. Now your heart is light and your 'cup runneth over' as your vibration raises.

Taking this time to learn about your body, to become more aware of your body, and awaken to who-you-really-are gifts you with the necessary tools to truly transform.

"Transformation literally means going beyond your form."

Wayne Dyer.

Being aware that finding lightness is not simply a physical journey, but an emotional one too has the potential for you to find not just lightness but peace in your skin. Becoming more conscious of what you are consuming through energy, thoughts, emotions and food, is your next evolutionary step within the realms of diet, health and wellbeing.

"And the day came when the risk it took to remain tight in the bud was more painful than the risk it took to blossom."

Anais Nin

Chakra's - Connecting the Dots!

I've mentioned 'energy' a lot, so let's take a look at the energy system, connecting the dots relative to your wellbeing and feeling lighter.

It took me a while to realize that everything in my body was connected, from my physical limbs and organs, to my thoughts, emotions and experiences. But when I did, it was the beginning of me finally understanding how I could effectively change and influence my body, and this marked the moving beyond fear, anxiety and confusion!

Everyone seems to have a theory, or explanation, of the chakra system, what it is and what it isn't. The trick is to not get too specific or intellectual about the whole thing, but rather, have a general appreciation of your energy system to put everything I have been talking about into perspective.

OK, just like your digestive system moves nutrients around your body, your cardiovascular moves blood, your lymphatic moves fluids, your endocrine moves hormones, your chakra system moves energy and this energy feeds every other system in your body, it is like the circuit board which powers everything else, literally circulating life force energy around your body.

Essentially the chakra system is an energy network, imagine highways and junctions that your life force uses to flow around your body. Within this network, we have seven major areas of interest where the energy congregates and creates almost a vortex like, spinning wheel of energy that provides nourishment for your physical organs that are in its vicinity. In this sense each chakra serves a purpose, associated with specific parts of our body in a very physical sense, but also in an emotional one too. Therefore our chakra system is an intrinsic part of our body as it facilitates the consciousness that we are into physical form, breathing life from the non-physical into the physical, and this is why it is essential to have an understanding of this whenever you are addressing your body, for health or weight, it is the basis from which all else springs.

There are seven major chakras in your body, staring from the Root Chakra, located at your pubic bone, traveling up through your body to your Crown Chakra above your head. The first chakra, the Root, governs desire, survival, vitality, and individuality. The second chakra is just below the navel and is referred to as the Sacral Chakra. This is the emotion center, where we experience, or feel rather, our instant feelings about something. This area is all about creation, fertility, nourishment and support. Therefore, our ability to take nourishment from food and experiences is determined by the energy here in the Sacral Chakra, which feeds the Spleen, the organ I explained earlier was responsible for our ability to absorb nourishment and feel comforted. This is why we have the link between food and emotional eating, it is all happening in this same area!

The third chakra is found just above the navel and is called the Solar Plexus Chakra, our inner sunshine, where our personal power is and also our digestive fires, since the Solar Plexus governs the stomach, liver and digestion. Our digestion of life and ability to process what we experience is embedded in this energy center.

The fourth chakra is at our heart, the Heart Chakra, and is the major feeling/emotional center. It's also the gateway to the non-physical realms, helping to free us from being entirely physically focused. If the energy here doesn't move in a healthy way then we feel sad, depressed, lacking faith as we solely focus on the physical rather than appreciating All that is, lacking love for who-we-really-are and becoming isolated rather than connected, fear filled rather than love filled.

From here, we go to the Throat Chakra, the Brow Chakra and Crown Chakra. These are the more non-physical aspects of our Being, concerning the power of our thoughts, intuition, imagination and greater connection to the universe. Here we have totally transformed our focus and approach to our body as we embrace and use the power of our thoughts, realizing that we do indeed create our own reality. Here is freedom from the confines of a purely physically focused life, and in this expanded awareness we find greater, more powerful tools, in the creation of our physical manifestation, which is what I have been explaining to you throughout this book, and what I integrate in this 8 week experience of creating your most BeUtiful Body!

Knowing all of this means that we cannot go back to our old diet ways of starving ourselves and calorie counting. There is absolutely no reason why we should not be integrating all of this wisdom into the pursuit of our own BeUtiful Body, and this is exactly what we are going to do now!

Part 6 - Get BeUtiful Body Ready

Get Ready

Remember this moment because it is pivotal. You are about to make a different choice from those you have been making about food and your body for your entire life up to this point. Now, you are different, you know more than you did before you started reading this book, now you know that it's all about love. Now, you are in a powerful place to make a change, to choose self-love and self-care, because you know that your life, your peace of mind, your wellbeing, your health and your most BeUtiful body all depend upon your ability to choose love over fear.

It is time to get ready! Ready to feel light, ready to feel beautiful, ready to digest your food with ease and this means starting from a place of love and cultivating the necessary inner environment that will allow all of this to happen, naturally. Everything is vibration, first and foremost, so you need to get yourself 'ready' by working with your vibration before you do anything else. Are you ready to get ready? Oh yes! Here goes, you need to get yourself connected!

Get Connected

From this moment, your top priority is to connect more deeply with U. This has to be your top priority because if you are not fully connected then feeling the love for yourself is definitely hard work and knowing what to eat to create more balance becomes impossible. It's a daily commitment, sometimes hourly, sometimes moment by moment even, depending on what's going on around you! But when I do this, life feels so much easier, there is a flow and a rhythm, even amidst uncertainty, that gives me a level of ease and grace that permeates through my entire body. You cannot be scrambled and chaotic in your energy and mind, and expect your body to look like a beautifully balanced, light, and graceful creation.

Remember, stress creates a heavy mind which creates a heavy body, peace creates a light mind, which means a light body! You get to choose your 'state' and this choice is the most powerful one you will ever make. The best part about it all is that the more you get connected with U the easier everything becomes, including feeling lighter!

To do this you have got to make the journey from being stuck in your head, mentally figuring everything out, down into your body, grounding all your energy, to come comfortably into the present moment. This means sinking deeper into your heart, into your stomach, where all of your power is, in your Solar Plexus, this is your anchor, this is your stability, operating from here helps you to instinctively feel what is good for you and what isn't, and especially with food.

There is way too much thinking going on, and the problem with this is that we ironically trap ourselves within the same habits of thought that have caused the dis-ease in the first place.

"A consistent thinker is a thoughtless person, because he conforms to a pattern; he repeats phrases and thinks in a groove."

Jiddu Krishnamurti

You have to find a way to quiet your mind, to step out of the stream of chatter that rules you life and that informs your choices, you have to make space for a different way, and this means you have to free your mind from the constant negative, critical, judgmental noise and get into your body, where you heart and instincts can be heard.

"Only the free mind knows what Love is."

Jiddu Krishnamurti

I know, this can be a tough call, believe me, my mind runs at a thousand miles an hour and can wrestle the best of them to the ground. But you have to make the shift from being ran by your mind to you running your mind, based upon your conscious choices rooted in instinct and connection to yourself.

"The body benefits from movement, and the mind benefits from stillness."

Sakyong Mipham

With this in mind, here are my three essentials for getting more connected:

» *Be Still*

» *Move*

» *Be In Nature*

I integrate them on a daily basis, even now, they remain the foundation of my self-care practice and help me to feel, balanced, calm and clear. They have taken the place of mindless, almost tortuous, routines that I used to put myself through, and I can tell you, give me these three any day! The fact that they've directly contributed to creating a body that I am comfortable within is a bonus.

BE STILL

Meditation just has it going on! So before you skip a few pages, because I know that when you're uncomfortable in your skin, the last thing you want to do is be still in it, don't underestimate its simplicity. Even though I'm a nutritionist, passionate about the power of food, there is no amount of healthy eating and exercise that can heal and enlighten your body if you are otherwise in a state of frenzied chaos! You have to find a way of Being still.

There are so many different types of meditation, silent, with music, sitting, lying, singing, still, moving, etc. So many different schools on this, no one is any better than the other, you just have to find what feels good. My favorite is sitting eyes closed and focusing on my breath. Choose your style, then commit to a daily practice, in the morning is best I find, and aim for 15-20 minutes. Set a timer on your iPhone or download Insight Timer, an incredible meditation app that is free and has loads of different mediations on there as well as connecting a global community of meditators.

You have to get out of your head and into your heart, so your journey becomes one of love and peace instead of fear and stress. Meditation is a powerful tool to get you there.

The simplest things are the most powerful, with simplicity comes consistency, and something that you do daily, however small or seemingly insignificant, is infinitely more powerful than anything that you do occasionally.

> **"Watch your actions for they become habits, watch your habits for they become character, watch your character, it becomes your destiny."**
>
> *Lao Tzu*

When I consider all the things that I have learnt along my journey, this is the one thing that felt as if it 'saved' me from my mind. "Meditation, meditation, meditation", the words of my mum ringing through my ears for years. I was reluctant at best, totally resistant at worst, but the day came when I surrendered, sat down and took a breath.

When did you last take a breath that you were conscious of?

Don't let it be your last breath that gets your attention. The biggest tragedy would be to have been alive and to never have truly felt it, to be made of light and to never have really known it.

Take the time to explore different types of mediation and see what feels good for you, it is not how you do it, but that you commit daily time for yourself, this is how you heal, this is how you connect.

MOVE

> **"Yoga is the journey of the self, through the self, to the self."**
>
> *The Bhagavad Gita*

It is challenging to express in words the power and beauty of this practice, it is a lifestyle and it gave me a completely new way of interacting with my body that changed my entire world. I had come to yoga under duress, my body literally could not cope anymore with my old routine. I had been working out really hard, not eating enough and ignoring injuries. I was actually making myself weaker not stronger because of this, to the point where my body said "enough is enough" and I literally could not run, or do anything challenging, because I was in too much physical pain, my back, stomach, hip and knees, they were all screaming "no more"!

After a few weeks of forced non-activity, I was feeling irritated and bored, so I had the idea that perhaps yoga would be a bridge from where I was now to getting myself 'fit' for my old routine again. Yoga had other plans however, it was bridge, but to an entirely different place, and for that, I am deeply appreciative.

Yes, yoga has been a powerful tool of transformation for me and I believe it could be for you, too. But again, there are so many ways 'to move' and it's important that you find what feels good for you. Dance is another movement that is amazing for reconnecting and there are so many fun classes that you can join. Pilates, Tai Chi, or any type of movement that encourages an awareness of your breath and working with your body consciously. Swimming is amazing for helping you to connect with your breath and move in a harmonious way, walking is also one of my favourites.

Most of all you need to find something that you actually enjoy, that you look forward to because it feels good and your body loves it too. Don't settle for anything less because you won't sustain it. Give yourself the freedom to explore, to try something new, to dedicate time to looking around and finding a new class or a new way of moving your body that you love.

BE IN NATURE

Being in nature just feels good, it's uplifting, and definitely gets the blood and oxygen flowing! You don't need a study to tell you that, but there is compelling research that has now quantified the 'value' and benefits to our health, both physical and mental, of getting out in nature. This one particular study blew my mind, it found that strolling through nature for just 1.5 hours reduced the amount of negative thinking by half[25]! Imagine halving the number of negative thoughts you have about yourself, or your weight, today! I have been talking about the power of our thoughts in creating our reality and physical body, and the harm that negative thoughts cause, well, if you can reduce them by half just by getting out in nature then we all need to get out side, like now!

The Law of Resonance explains in part why getting out in nature would have such a beneficial impact on our state of being. This law states that "our life force will react to every stimulus, or force, that it is being exposed to. If the force of the stimulus is stronger that the inner life force present, the bodies are forced to adjust in a way where a consequence of that force is perceived or experienced.[26]" In physics, resonance is a "phenomenon in which a vibrating system or external force drives another system to oscillate with greater amplitude.[27]" We are vibrating energy, we live in a vibrational universe, and nature is vibrating too, so being out in it long enough effects our vibrational state and encourages our vibration to 'resonate' with it. So, when we put ourselves among the high vibration of nature it helps our vibration to rise in a way that awakens us to our nature. Get outside, stand amongst hills, trees, meadows, flowers, mountains, rivers, ocean or whatever you have around your area and open your eyes and see its beauty, absorb it, notice it, tune your senses to look for the beauty that surrounds you and know that this same nature which you are observing is exactly the same as you.

Add a good walk in there too and you have a recipe for a BeUtiful mind and body! This is one of my favorite ways to care for my body, and so much nicer than running, for me anyway. When I finally gave myself permission to walk rather than run most days, my body sighed with relief and let go of loads of heavy stress in the process!

The movement of walking massages internal organs, gets the lymphatic system moving, without causing stress on your system, and it moves energy, it gets you flowing! Good news for you feeling lighter.

Use this time to really get 'in' to your body, connect with it, feel it, and find your own rhythm. Try consciously breathing whilst you are walking, this feels incredible for me, I learnt the importance of this the hard way up in the Andes. Altitude sickness was such a pain for me but I found that as long as I didn't let myself get out of breath, if I consciously breathed deeply and slowly and only moved at a speed where I could maintain this steady flow, my body coped really well and I could keep going. Our bodies are capable of amazing things when we connect to them, pay attention, and act in alignment with them. This was a habit that I have continued, even when at sea level! Try it! It is actually incredibly empowering because you tap into your strength and endurance in a peaceful way, think of the lightness this allows!

Love your Body, Unconditionally

Now you're getting connected you need to amp up the love!

"Love your body? Yeah right", is the usual response when we are in the midst of body hating! I used to think, "how can I love my body when I don't even like it?" Two things wrong with this line of questioning and the premise upon which it is based. First, what is love? Second, what is my experience of love?

What is love? By asking the question 'how can I love my body' I'm actually missing the point completely. I AM love, so are you, LOVE is what we are, so my question is instantly separating myself from the love that I am already. We are an expression of love, since love is all there is, then it follows that everything is love, including you and me, and love is oneness, not separation. In realizing that we already are love, it now becomes more about our awareness of this rather than trying to 'get' it. No wonder love always feels so out of reach when we chase it under the false belief that we are not 'it' already. Love isn't something to conjure, it is something to become aware that we are.

What is my experience of love? Well, I have to admit, and I am sure you can relate to this too, our experience of our idea of 'love' isn't always feeling like champagne and chocolate moments. We kind of get the feeling that 'love' is somehow conditional, we please people and they seem to love us, we don't please them and they don't love us. This may or may not be accurate but it sure does feel like this, even within family and friends, our love relationships can be very dysfunctional leaving us out of love with love. But that really isn't what love is, like beauty, it isn't bound by conditions and limits. Love isn't fickle, despite many life experiences and relationships that may have taught us differently. The problem is, not only do we take these definitions and experiences of love with us to our loved ones, we take them to our Self and our body. Caught up in our own web of conditions and limits, holding on so tightly to these that there is no room for the light to enter.

Put the word 'unconditional' in front of love and something rather magical happens. Now you get to the essence of what 'love' really is. Thankfully, the closer you get to understanding it, the easier it becomes to feel it and to Be it, because it's unconditional!

No longer do you have to wait for a certain number on the scale before you can love your body, because real love is unconditional, you open up a window of opportunity to Be the love right now and your body will sigh such relief the moment you do. The ease, the releasing of tension in your tummy as you finally take a deep breath and let it all go because, whilst you may not have your idea of perfect hips, you can love your body regardless!

Why is this so important? Because beauty always comes from love, it can never ever come from a place of body hating. If you really want to feel and look beautiful, you have to love your body beautiful. There is no nutrient or food that can replace it, love for your body is what will set you free from dieting dramas and allow your body to feel the lightness that you are wanting. In fact, if you could find a way to bottle self-love there would be no need for any other medicine, it would be a cure all.

> *"Your task is not to seek for love, but merely to seek and find all the barriers within yourself that you have built against it."*
>
> *Rumi*

Ask yourself what it is that you don't love about your body, and I mean the real why. Not the surface 'why', because it looks like this or that. The deep rooted, what it represents to you, how it makes you feel, this sort of 'why'. When you bring conscious awareness to a deep rooted pain, negative belief or opinion, you also bring understanding. Over-time understanding brings compassion, with more time comes appreciation, because as you confront these issues you're shining light on them and slowly but surely they lose their power.

Love isn't something you have to magic out of thin air or figure out how to 'do'. It is what you are. And when you let go and unravel all the negative, fear based, beliefs and opinions, you're not left with nothing. What you are left with is love because it is what you are already. Through this process you've just found the barriers within yourself that you have built against it, and clearing these barriers automatically connects you to love.

I love 3's, so here we go for my body loving recipe to get us all in the mood right now because your body has been starved long enough:

» *Awareness*

» *Appreciation*

» *Acceptance*

Let's go through these one-by-one so you can start loving your body now, without anything having to physically change, just your own perception and focus.

AWARENESS

Know thyself. Know your body, because all negativity is born from ignorance. Being so caught up in all the surface stuff, like what your body weighs, has left you completely oblivious to the magic that is happening within your body, right under your nose, in every single moment.

By getting to know your body, your perspective and awareness of how intelligent and incredible it is will expand exponentially, as you become increasingly aware of the genius within, keeping your heart beating and lungs breathing.

Take a deep breath, exhale fully and remind yourself, daily, of how amazing your body is;

Your body is Amazing

Your body is an amazing feat of evolutionary genius, it serves you to the best of its ability, every single day, keeping you alive, even whilst you sleep, breathing vital life force without you even having to think about it.

Your body is Genius

That breath fuels complex systems that not only allow your body to function, but to self-heal. Your body has the ability to renew itself, at a cellular level, every seven years. Clearing away all the negativity and toxicity whilst embracing the nourishment and love so it can survive and thrive.

Your Body is your Best Friend

Your body goes everywhere with you, willingly supporting you, as much as you allow, through your entire physical life, and it does so unconditionally. In this moment you have breath in your lungs, and so, all things are possible.

Pause for a moment. Open your BeUtiful Body journal and write down your feelings to these questions:

» *How did these words make you feel?*

» *Did it spark a sense of knowing within you?*

» *Do you feel any sense of relief or lightness when you read these words?*

Go back and re-read this passage, breathing deeply, consciously feeding yourself with this body wisdom. Read it whenever you find yourself slipping into old thought patterns of body shaming and replace those thoughts with this greater awareness.

Self-Love Practice - Please keep this passage close to your bed and read it every night before you go to sleep, not only will this help you to begin looking at your body with greater awareness, it will naturally pave the way for our next step of appreciation.

APPRECIATION

Greater awareness leads us naturally into the second step of appreciation.

Appreciation sounds so gentle and yet it is one of the most powerful emotions you can feel when it comes to attracting what you want. I know, it is the last thing you want to do when you feel so unhappy with your body, but you cannot Be light if you feel heavy. You cannot be beautiful, at least through your eyes and those are the only eyes that matter, if you are feeling negative about your body.

Appreciation is a game changer because your body wants to be loved and appreciated, it doesn't want to be hated and shamed.

Love and appreciation helps your body to relax whilst hating creates stress and disharmony. Looking in the mirror and thinking how fat your thighs look will not make them thin, I have tried, many times, they won't budge, even a millimeter. However, appreciating them for allowing you to walk and exercise, whilst finding other parts of your body that you can feel appreciation for will!

Self-Love Practice - Get your BeUtiful Body journal and write five things that you feel appreciation for about your body. List them, just one word answers if that's all you've got for now. Let this become a daily practice, if you want your physical body to change on the outside then you must change what's happening on the inside first.

ACCEPTANCE

This is a big one, and it is the launching pad for all positive transformation. Acceptance of your body is the final release of struggle and stress making way for ease and peace. Your body will breathe a huge sigh of relief and let all the angst, pent up negativity, and disappointment out when you finally accept what is.

This isn't to say that in your acceptance you're 'making do' with what you have and succumbing to it without any window of change. Absolutely not. The total opposite is true.

In accepting your body, you are putting yourself in the perfect place to create exactly what it is you want, because for the first time, you are starting from a place of ease and love rather than struggling to get away from something you don't like or are fearful of. In fact, struggling against anything will ensure that it stays!

Your body is constantly forming and then reforming, in every instance you have the opportunity to actively effect this reformation into a form that you desire through the power of thought and the power of food. If you do not change what you feed those new cells on a physical, mental, emotional and spiritual level, then your body will not be able to change.

It is with acceptance that you allow this continual death and rebirth to be a positive progression, rather than simply repeating what is already. In your acceptance of your body, you create the necessary environment for different intelligence to inform each and every one of your cells and create the body you want.

Affirming to yourself 'I accept my body, just the way it is now, and I love my body unconditionally,' is a powerful statement. Write this down in your BeUtiful Body journal, say it to yourself, remind yourself of this whenever negative thoughts creep in.

There is no magic bullet to this, it is a day to day choice. You can either continue to think harmful thoughts and hate your body or you can decide enough is enough and accept your body the way that it is.

Self-Love Practice - Remember the scene in Bridget Jones where Mr. Darcy tells her that he loves her, just the way she is? I want you to channel these vibes for your body, accepting your body, just as it is now, and writing this down in your BeUtiful Body journal every single night, "I accept my body, just the way it is now." Give your body the gift of your own unconditional love and notice the difference this makes. Self-love is a game changer.

Free Your Mind

I was walking on the treadmill one day, avoiding the fierce heat of a Dubai summer. Catching a glimpse of myself in the mirrors, I noticed how easy it was for me to slip into thinking about myself and my body in a negative way. It is really quite amazing how powerful our beliefs are, and how a label, or diagnosis, seems to stick like super-glue!

To give you a personal example. For years, since I was 16, I felt my hormones were a problem, never managing to feel balanced and experienced a wrath of symptoms as a result. That day on the treadmill, I thought to myself, "what if I am limiting myself, what if my constant judgement and belief that my hormones are unbalanced, is preventing them from coming into balance? What if I was the saboteur, perpetuating the imbalance?"

I realized in that moment that I had to find a way to let go of my 'belief' and constant inner dialogue telling myself that my hormones were a problem and always out of balance. Perhaps they had been out of balance and needed my help, but this 'help' must also come in the form of me letting go of this belief to allow balance to be found. In my hastiness to always 'blame' them, perhaps what I thought was 'imbalance' and something 'wrong' wasn't at all, just my body trying to get my attention.

From that day I consciously decided not to allow that habitual dialogue to run through my mind. I stopped telling myself that story. Every time I caught myself reverting back to that old story I stopped the thoughts and refocused them onto "my body is intelligent, I appreciate the wisdom it shares with me, the more I relax and find ease the more my body comes into balance and the happier my hormones become and I know that my body and hormones know exactly how to do that, and if they need my help I trust I will be intuitively drawn to whatever is needed."

This is still something I am working with today, but I have already felt the physical improvement. Those habitual old stories still pop into my head from time to time, but every time they do there is an opportunity for me to practice self-love and care.

Creating something new relies on your ability to tell a new story, and daily mantras can be an excellent way of training your mind to focus the way you want it to. If you don't, your mind is like an elastic band that can only go so far but will always ping back to your default stories.

Mantra Magic

Replacing negative dialogue with a little mantra magic works wonders for helping you to feel more positive and love focused. Energy follows thought, as you direct your thoughts you direct your energy, and this forms a powerful intention that has the ability to transform your body.

These are some of my favorite mantras, but you can make up your own that feel meaningful for you. I find it helps to write them down, and even say them to myself. What is important is that you have something positive to replace negative thoughts with.

My favorite Mantras:

- » *I digest food with ease*

- » *My body comfortably absorbs all the love and nourishment it needs from food*

- » *I choose to eat food that I love and that loves my body*

- » *My most natural state is light and healthy*

» *All the cells in my body are happy and work in harmony*

» *It is easy for my body to feel light*

Your Mantra Practice - Get your BeUtiful Body journal and begin writing one of my mantras down and see how that feels for you. Now start to craft your own, be simple, be easy, don't make them too difficult for you to believe, this is the secret to a mantra, you have to believe it, if you can't believe it yet then start with something easier, or more general. Once you have two or three mantras that resonate with you, read them daily, and repeat them to yourself throughout the day to keep positively directing your thoughts and energy.

Intuitive Eating & Body Wisdom

This is how you put love for food, your body and yourself into practice. This goes beyond just being conscious of eating a relatively healthy diet, and factors your unique body into the equation. This is the primary intention of body wisdom led nutrition, to eat in a way that honors you, that nourishes and nurtures your body, that reconnects you with your true nature, loving the food you eat and eating the food that loves you back.

Intuitive Eater Practice - This practice is all about coming into the moment and feeling where you and your body are, physically and emotionally. If you check-in with yourself, you will be in the best place to make a choice about food that will heal rather than harm, that will create lightness rather than heaviness. Try not to sensor your thoughts with what you think you should be eating, instead, give your body freedom to inspire you with its wisdom. Each time you notice that you are hungry, ask yourself these questions before you 'just eat something', and remember, first and foremost, food is vibrational energy:

» *You're hungry, how hungry?*

» *Are you hungry for food or something else?*

» *If it is food, what do you really fancy and why?*

» *Is it your body that would love to eat this food, or is this food something you think you should be eating?*

» *If you're not hungry for food, what are you hungry for?*

» *Breathe deeply and ask your body what it would most love to eat? Something warm or cold, comforting or fresh, spicy or cooling, cooked or raw, sweet or savory, moist or dry? Think about colors, flavors, textures and tastes - like in Ayurveda. The list is endless, but keep asking until you get a feel for what would most nourish your body in this moment.*

» *Whilst eating, ask yourself, does it taste good? Is it pleasurable and are you allowing yourself to receive the pleasure within this food?*

» *You've finished eating, how do you feel now? Full, too full, still hungry, comfortable, irritated, heavy, light, happy, guilty?*

This is a practice to take with you to each meal and snack. Checking-in with your body and using your body wisdom and guidance to help you to decide what to eat. When we go through the upcoming 8 week process together, keep this practice going, don't just blindly follow what I have written for that week. Yes, use my menus and suggestions as inspiration, but you must always follow your body wisdom and build your connection with yourself. Never let this go!

However, you can only eat intuitively if you are conscious of your body wisdom, so here is a practice to help strengthen your ability to hear your body wisdom and, most importantly, act upon it!

Body Wisdom Practice - This is very similar to the Intuitive Eating Practice, but a retrospective exercise for the end of the day to strengthen your conscious awareness and nurture your intuitively knowing, all of which is going to build trust, in yourself!

» *Begin this evening, in your BeUtiful Body journal, make a note of all that you have eaten today, not for the purpose of nit picking through it, but to understand how your body responds to certain foods.*

» *Once you have listed the foods, then make a note of how you felt today, did you experience bloating, constipation, diarrhea, wind, gas, lethargy, headaches etc? Did you feel energized or exhausted, how did you sleep the night before? Write down all things that come to mind.*

» *Now, glance back over your foods and see if anything jumps out at you for being 'contributing factors', to any of the symptoms you noted down, positive or negative. After a few days a pattern may begin to emerge so keep looking back over the previous days and see what is really going on for you. Please keep in mind that the same foods may have differing impacts based upon how you cook them, what you eat them with, what time of day you eat them and your emotional state. For example, a coffee may well be perfect one day, but then on another day, if you're feeling really stressed and emotional, the coffee may just tip you over the edge and make you feel terrible! You can't text book this, you have to connect with yourself and notice what is true for your body!*

» *Now, once you recognize a food, group of foods or mode of cooking that repeatedly contributes to you not feeling good, physically, mentally or emotionally, then make the conscious choice to not eat that food, in that combination or way of cooking, for a period of 8-12 weeks, to give your body a complete rest. Or, if you notice a pattern between your emotional state and foods that leaves you feeling awful, then make a conscious choice to not repeat that combination again. For example, don't have a coffee if you're feeling super emotional! As you streamline your eating, relative to your unique body, you will very quickly feel your body come into balance and feel lighter.*

Part 7 - Your BeUtiful Body

You Are Ready!

But before you go diving into the first smoothie bowl, just remember, this is not a diet plan for you to mindlessly follow, this is a process of using food to heal your body and encourage lightness, so keep your Intuitive Eating and Body Wisdom practices up.

Also, keep reminding yourself of all that you now know, each time an old diet thought comes into your mind, consciously choose to focus your thoughts, remembering your self-love practices and all that we have been talking about.

It is OK if you have body negative thoughts and anxious moments, it took me a while to get used to eating with love, and it felt so strange to not have guilty feelings after every meal. I realized I had fallen into the trap of almost having to feel guilty after eating just to satisfy myself that I wasn't eating recklessly, and to keep myself in-check.

It had become a habit! When I first moved into a more love filled mindset, it felt so weird, as if I had I lost a part of my identity. I felt like I was reacquainting myself, with myself, it sounds weird but then one day it suddenly hit me, I was literally learning how to eat and nourish myself, on all levels, because I had no idea how to eat without being on a diet! And, I'd had no idea of who I really was, or rather, what I am.

It took time to train my thoughts toward the positive aspects of food and why I was eating, my old negative thoughts would hijack me at the most unsuspecting times, but after a while these became less and less. It is a process so be gentle with yourself, but most of all, be conscious of whatever is in your mind because you cannot change what you are not conscious of.

If you do get moments of diet crisis, take a moment to breathe, put your hands on your tummy and feel your breath. Observe the thoughts you are having, and then softly remind yourself of All that you now know.

Here is what your 8 week journey to create your most BeUtiful body looks like -

Week 1 - Lighten Up

Say "no" to foods that harm, and "yes" to foods that love U!.

Week 2 - Burn Baby Burn

Rekindle your digestive fire and ignite your transformational power.

Week 3 - Be Calm & Connect

Calming, connecting and soothing body, mind and soul.

Week 4 - Feel Nourished

Diving deep into your well of Being and nourishing your spleen so you can feel the LOVE.

Week 5 - BeU Ritual; Rest & Digest

A powerful 3 day ritual to rest and revive your digestion for a lighter feeling body.

Week 6 - Let Go

Going, going, gone! Cleansing toxins, physical and emotional, as we energize your liver.

Week 7 - BeU Ritual; Love & Light

A beautiful 3 day ritual to bring you into your heart.

Week 8 - Be Light

Believe and you will see!

Extra weekly guidance and all supporting notes and recipes you can find on my website - www.lovebeu.com.

This is a process, a journey, one that's never ending because there is no end to U. Please read each week first and then come back to week 1 and begin the process in your own time.

During each week I ask you to check in with how your body reacts and choose which advice and inspiration you follow, and which you do not. Remember, there is no one size fits all! However, the essence is constant, so you will be able to choose within all of this what feels good for you and your body, and you must allow yourself the freedom to do just that, this is your journey!

Also, the following weeks are a continuation of each other, adding to and building upon rather than a 'do this and now do that' approach.

The aim is to eventually incorporate the essence of all 8 weeks into your eating and caring for your body, in a way that your body wants and at a time when it needs it most. You will learn exactly what that means as you go through this process, so, with an open mind and open heart, here we go.

Week 1 - Lighten Up

BeUtiful Mantra - I am ready to lighten up and practice self-love through what I eat and what I think.

Part of using food as a tool of self-love rather than harm is consciously choosing not to feed your body with foods that you already know do not feel good to eat. Bloating, heaviness, lethargy, and all other digestive disturbances, are not how you should feel after eating. If you do, then this is your body trying to let you know that it doesn't like it.

You also need to start making your body's processes function as easy and efficiently as possible to start feeling lighter, so I have have included practical suggestions of how to eat and what to eat to create more ease in your body, especially for your digestion.

Time to lighten the load now! Here's this weeks guidance for you to follow and integrate into your daily routine:

Consciously Connect With Your Body - Do not leave yourself even for one meal! From this moment I want you to stay with yourself no matter what. Be conscious and honest with yourself of which foods feel good and which foods don't. Keep up your BeUtiful Body journal, noting what you've eaten and how it made you feel.

Food LOVE Not HARM - Listen to your body wisdom and all this information you receive from your body and act, or rather, eat accordingly! Do not eat something that you know is going to make you feel bloated or lethargic. Just don't, choose self-love, not harm, at each and every mealtime.

Hydrate - Water is vital if you want to feel lighter and reduce your toxicity. Drink water evenly and consistency throughout the day, being careful not to gulp it down in one go, this will just make you feel bloated and heavy. There is no universal amount of water that is right for everybody, so pay attention to your body. As a guide, aim for at least 2 liters of pure, room temperature, mineral water daily. If you really want to get lighter and get things moving, drink 1 liter of water before breakfast!

Eat Natural - As much as possible, avoid processed food products, especially those with ingredients that you can't read. Be conscious of what you are putting into your body, read the ingredients list on the food and then decide if you still want to eat it. Inform yourself and make empowered food choices.

Limit Dairy, Wheat, and Sugar - Yes, right now, because these foods are most often the usual suspects of digestive disturbances and create all sorts of problems in your body! Even if you do not have any major digestive issues it is still worth limiting them and noticing the difference you feel in your body. And, they are low vibration foods, and you just don't need heavy vibes clogging up your body if you want to feel lighter!

Only Eat Fruit on an Empty Stomach - Fruit takes very little time to digest so if you have a stomach full of food it sits on top of that and begins to putrefy causing toxins and gas. Only ever eat fruit on an empty stomach, at breakfast for example, or 2 hours since you last ate something. Never eat fruit as a dessert, from a digestive standpoint you are better off with dark chocolate!

Eat Plants - Consciously direct your eating to a more plant based diet. This is kinder for your body, kinder for the environment, and easier for your body to digest. I'm not asking you to become vegan, I'm wanting you to 'Be U', and as far as food is concerned, eating more plant based foods raises your vibration and makes connecting with who-you-really-are a much easier process.

Week 2 - Burn Baby Burn

BeUtiful Mantra - I digest food, emotions and thoughts with ease, and I naturally feel lighter.

What you eat is important, but how you eat is just as significant, especially when it comes to rekindling your digestion. The truth is, if you get the 'how' part right and you've successfully managed to 'lighten the load', then you are really buying yourself so much leeway with your eating, because you're doing it in a way that is in tune with your body!

The all-important HOW to Eat

Now that we are in the process of lightening the load, I want you to follow these 'how to' rules of eating. Whatever you are eating, eat it like this -

Timing - Don't eat when you are stressed, emotional, or in a hurry. Your digestive system doesn't work well under these conditions and causes indigestion, bloating and heaviness. Make time to eat and sit calmly, focusing on what you are putting into your body. This does take discipline but try to gift yourself the time to mindfully eat your meals. If you are emotional or stressed then at least consciously calm your system down before eating by sitting quietly and breathing deeply for 3-5 minutes. Simple but effective, so don't knock it until you've tried it!

Routine & Consistency - Your body thrives on routine and consistency, your spleen does too. This is what will allow your digestion to relax and regulate your entire system. When you eat and sleep sporadically, this creates uncertainty, your body, especially your digestion, doesn't tolerate uncertainty well and it causes stress. This also disrupts your hormonal balance and appetite, making weight extra difficult to address. As you go through this week create your own daily routine, and do your best to practice it every day, sleeping and eating at regular and convenient times, and particularly don't go too long without eating. Don't let your body feel like you've abandoned it!

We can't 'burn baby burn' without some specific digestive miracle working tips! As you feel inspired, start to incorporate these tips to get everything moving so you can feel lighter. Their power is in consistency, so build them into your daily routine for optimal benefits:

Probiotics - Supporting your gut flora is such a powerful way to improve your health and feel lighter. In Ayurveda, all dis-ease is rooted in poor digestion, too often our digestive systems are compromised and under toxic load, whether that be from food intolerances, undiagnosed allergies, poor eating habits, stress, lifestyle factors or medications like antibiotics, which damage your vital gut flora. Start taking a good quality probiotic, experiment with different brands until you find one that feels good for you.

Prebiotics - Helping to feed probiotics in your stomach, prebiotics enhance your overall gut flora and play a vital role in your digestion.

Often under-appreciated, prebiotics are really important in maintaining digestive health, and therefore helping you to feel lighter. Prebiotics are found in raw garlic, artichokes, onions and dandelion greens, raw leeks, raw asparagus and raw chicory root. Mindfully incorporate more of these foods into your daily eating in a way that feels good for your body.

Enhance Your Stomach Acid - Stomach acid levels are super important for your digestion, this is why taking antacids for indigestion just makes your digestion worse, as often, it is insufficient stomach acid that is causing the problem not too much. If you don't have sufficient stomach acid then you can't break down what you eat, this makes feeling lighter almost impossible. You can enhance your stomach acid very simply by drinking water and freshly squeezed lemon juice between meals, or by blending 1-2 teaspoons of raw apple cider vinegar with a cup of warm water and drinking daily in the morning or before meals.

Fresh Ginger - Incorporate more fresh ginger into your food. My favourite way to do this is to blend a 1-2cm piece of fresh raw ginger root in a smoothie. Or you can use in cooking, like a stir-fry, or make fresh ginger tea. Ginger encourages digestive fire whilst helping to get rid of toxicity in the stomach and any undigested foods.

Always Chew Food Properly - Your stomach doesn't have teeth, so if you don't chew your food your stomach gets filled with chucks of food that it cannot break down properly, this definitely causes unwanted heaviness. "A well chewed burger is better than a badly chewed salad for your waist line." Dr. Harold Stossier.

Don't Ignore Hunger - So many times we have been taught to do this and it is an absolute disaster for digestion, often creating a lot of bloating and a slower metabolism. Listen to your body, eat when your body is asking for food, and try not to go more than four hours without eating.

Week 3 - Be Calm & Connect

BeUtiful Mantra - I am safe, I am secure in my body, I feel balanced and grounded and choose to eat in a way that helps me to feel this way.

To feel lighter you have to calm your body down first. Adrenal fatigue, caused by excessive stress, is one of the main reasons why it can feel difficult to lose weight, despite a clean diet and lots of exercise. In fact, if your system is over stressed and your adrenal glands are compromised, exercise can have the complete opposite effect, making you heavier and more bloated. In these cases, you have to slow down, calm down and give your body a chance to find its balance first, otherwise you will always feel heavy, regardless of how little you eat or how active you are! So this week is all about calming down, slowing down, reducing stress and anxiousness, so you can more easily feel balanced and connected.

This week I would like you to focus on the following steps to reduce stress, support your adrenal function and feel more balanced:

You Must Eat - Everyday, breakfast, lunch and dinner. This will help you to remain balanced, physically and emotionally, whilst supporting your metabolism and adrenal glands. Skipping meals, or going too long between eating, creates huge swings in blood sugar that negatively impacts your ability to remain calm and balanced, whilst damaging your metabolism, and creating stress. The absolutely worst meal to skip is lunch! This is when your digestion is at its strongest and your body needs food to literally anchor it, creating stability, energy and balance.

Stress Release - Remember those three ways to flush stress hormones from your tissues, rebounding, self-massage and orgasm? Hopefully you had already started to incorporate them into your self-care practice, if you haven't then start this week. Your body needs all the help it can get to eliminate the negative effects of stress hormones accumulating in your system.

Magnesium - The mineral of relaxation and often seriously deficient in a lot of people. Magnesium helps to harmonize pH balance, relieves stress and tension, soothes achy muscles and joints, lowers blood pressure, calms the central nervous system, balances hormones and aids in many other systems in your body. Eat raw cacao, spirulina powder, dark leafy greens, avocado, almonds, figs and pumpkin seeds. You can also use magnesium spray that you use directly onto your skin, this is also great to ease physical aches, pains and tension. Or, liquid nano-particle magnesium is my favorite way to supplement with this mineral. Bathing in epsom salts, which are magnesium, twice weekly for 20 minutes is an efficient use of time! You get your magnesium, it's restful, it eases stress and tension whilst aiding detoxification and harmonizing your pH levels. I use 4 tbsp of epsom salts per bath.

Rest - Sounds easy enough, but this is the one thing that is always lacking in busy lifestyles. If you are tired, listen to your body, don't drink coffee or eat sugar to keep going, stop! Rest heals. If you spend an hour taking your body to your physical limits through exercise, then you need to spend time taking your body to the opposite end of the spectrum to relaxation, this will also help your body to more positively respond to exercise! Take time to consciously relax, whether that be a bath, meditation, a yin yoga class or a nap, and notice how much lighter your body begins to feel. If time is short then cut back on your time spent exercising and invest this time into relaxing your mind and body. Yes, really!

Adrenal Stressors - Reduce as much as possible caffeine, sugar and alcohol. All of these trigger a stress response in your body and can over stimulate your system causing harm, particularly to your adrenal glands.

For The Love of God, Eat Carbohydrates - Do not cut these completely from your diet. Start eating nutrient rich complex carbohydrates like wild rice, brown rice, buckwheat, gluten-free oats, quinoa, root vegetables, beans and lentils. They will help you to feel more grounded and balanced whilst supporting your adrenal glands, and providing your body with vital nutrients and an efficient source of energy.

Ashwagandha - This is an adaptogenic herb that is popular in Ayurveda and plays a role in supporting both adrenal and thyroid function. You can get this from a good nutrition store, if this feels right for you then seek advice from a practitioner before supplementing. My favourite way to take ashwagandha is in powder form and I make a Blissful Tonic to soothe my adrenal glands;

Whisk together 1/2 teaspoon of ashwagandha powder, 1/2-2/3 cup of warmed nut milk (homemade milk makes this even nicer), 1/2 tsp cinnamon powder and a teaspoon of raw honey. Sip early in the morning, I usually have it before breakfast.

Holy Basil - One of the most sacred plants in India, and more commonly known as Tulsi. In Hindu mythology Tulsi symbolizes the goddess Lakshmi, representing abundance and beauty. This herb has been valued for centuries because of its incredible benefits for body, mind and spirit. Used for a variety of reasons, from common cold treatment to digestive issues, Holy Basil is an incredible adaptogenic plant. However, the most compelling area of its expertise, of which modern data and research is supporting, is its ability to reduce stress hormones, particularly corticosterone[28] that has been linked to greater mental clarity, improved memory and a reduced risk of age-related mental disorders. To get Holy Basil in your life start drinking Tulsi tea, find an organic, good quality brand from your local health store, and drink daily. You can also take supplemented forms of Holy Basil, just check with your practitioner before you start.

Week 4 - Feel Nourished

BeUtiful Mantra - I consciously choose to nourish myself with food and thoughts that help me to feel good.

This week is going to strengthen your spleen energy, helping you to feel grounded and nourished. This will help you to feel stronger and more content, physically and emotionally, and better able to practice self-love whilst positively addressing emotional eating.

Feel nourished by following this weeks guidance:

Food Color Healing - The color orange is associated with the sacral chakra, the spleen and helping you to feel nourished. This week incorporate foods like squash, pumpkin, sweet potato, carrots, mango, and papaya for example. Your spleen also loves yellow split peas, lentils, parsnips, and other root vegetables, oats, brown rice, and quinoa

Limit Cold Raw Foods - Salads, vegetable juices, fruit juices and raw vegetables, all tend to compromise the spleen if there is a preexisting weakness, and can cause bloating and digestive problems if your spleen energy is insufficient. Notice that I don't say avoid completely, just try not to fill your stomach with cold, wet juices and salads every breakfast, lunch and dinner. A great way of balancing this is to keep your raw food to the early part of the day and avoiding them late afternoon and evening, this will be working with your natural digestive rhythm and is helpful for a light feeling tummy.

Feel Cosy - Warming soups, casseroles, curries, stews, stir-fry's, roasted vegetables and steamed vegetables, especially in the evening help you to feel comforted and cosy. Warm food is also more satisfying, makes you feel fuller and more content, physically and emotionally. Instead of raw food in the evening try to have warm foods to nourish your spleen energy, this will be easier on your digestion too.

Plant Based Days - Try to have at least 3 plant based, vegan days per week, if you are not exclusively vegan/vegetarian already. This will help your digestion, reduce the toxic load on your system, encourage a higher vibration and supply more vital life force energy.

To help you with this week, I have put together a menu that you can use for inspiration. You don't need to be eating papaya and quinoa exclusively, just use this menu as a guide and practice eating intuitively. Be aware of how you feel when you are eating and what happens afterwards. Notice if a food feels good for you, if it doesn't make a note and don't eat it again.

This Week's Foodie Inspiration

(see www.lovebeu.com for all recipes)

Breakfast:

Quinoa & Cardamom Porridge with Apricots & Coconut Cream

Be Nurtured Mango Smoothie

Papaya Chia Seed Pudding

Lunch:

Comforting Grains & Greens Salad

Be Grounded Root Vegetable Soup

Cosy Split Pea Soup

Dinner:

Sweet Potato & Kale Coconut Curry

Roasted Root Vegetables with Rosemary & Feta Cheese

Sweet Potato Wedges & Melted Goats Cheese, with Mustard & Watercress

Week 5 - BeU Ritual; Rest & Digest

BeUtiful Mantra - When I give myself time to rest I can digest my food, thoughts, and emotions with greater ease and I feel lighter, naturally.

We are over half way so this is a good time to check-in with your digestion and help it to heal more deeply with a specific ritual to encourage your fire of transformation to burn brighter.

You will need three days for this, so try to find a little time when your week is at its quietest, to give your body the best chance to receive the benefits without you being rushed off your feet. If this doesn't quite fit with your diary, please don't worry and don't' rush this. Take your time and continue with the previous weeks until you are able to complete this.

These three days are all about resting your digestion, a simple but powerful process. Based on Ayurvedic principles, this healing ritual helps your body to reset your digestive system and enjoy a rest from foods that are difficult to break down, have toxins and chemicals in them and stimulants like sugar, caffeine, and alcohol.

Choose three consecutive days when work is at a minimum, there are no hardcore gym workouts, stressful meetings, deadlines, or anything that causes you to spend large amounts of energy, this is a time for rest…

Rest & Digest Ritual

(see www.lovebeu.com for all recipes)

On waking: Large mug of hot water with a slice of fresh ginger root

Breakfast: Peaceful Oats

Lunch (ideally 12noon-1pm): Restful Kitcheree

Dinner (ideally between 5-6pm): Restful Kitcheree

Night Time Tipple: Golden Mylk (if you feel you need)

Stay well hydrated, drinking up to 3 liters of room temperature, pure mineral water.

Daily Guidance

As you move through this three day ritual, eating the food listed above, please follow this daily guidance:

Day 1 - Rest your body

When you wake, before getting out of bed, take a moment to contemplate and remind yourself of the ritual you are undertaking for these next three days. Before you get up, laying comfortably in your bed, bring your attention to your breath, take long slow inhales and full exhales. How you start a day sets a precedent for what is to come, now gently set an intention for this first day, whatever feels most appropriate to you. When you feel ready, get up.

Drink hot water as you ease yourself into your first day of the ritual, maybe light an incense stick or a candle. Focus on taking little sips of your water, mindfully cleansing your body with this clean and pure water, thank it for being so gentle on your body and honor the intelligence held within the water cleansing and hydrating your body. Be conscious of your breathing, calm and full breaths, sit there peacefully whilst you finish your water.

Bring your intention to mind, think about your intention and keep it in your thoughts throughout the day.

Body brushing and a five minute self-massage would be wonderful if you have time to add to your usual morning routine.

For today, and the next two days, the food you eat will be simple and easy to digest. Be mindful when you eat, eat slower than you usually would to help your digestion do what it needs to. Eat dinner before 6pm and try not to eat anything after that, just warm water, herbal tea or golden mylk.

Get to bed early, take your BeUtiful Body journal with you, and write how you have felt today. Now ask your inner self if there is anything that it would like you to know? Write this question down and see if your pen continues writing an answer, relax your mind and enjoy this restful energy.

Thank your body for helping you through this day and now set an intention to rest deeply as you sleep.

Day 2 - Rest your Mind

As you wake, be gentle with yourself, notice how you feel and take a few moments like you did yesterday. Breathe mindfully, slowly, and deeply as you remind yourself of your intention for this ritual.

Hot water and ginger time with your favorite candle or incense. As you finish your water, stay here a few moments longer. Close your eyes, try to sit with your back straight but comfortable, lay the backs of your hands on your thighs and listen to your breath. Let this sound of your own breath guide you into a deeper state of relaxation and rest. It doesn't matter if thoughts come to mind, let them come and go. After five or ten minutes, or whenever you feel ready, gently open your eyes and take a big stretch…

If you can body brush and self-massage, then give yourself some time to do so.

Before you eat today, take a moment to appreciate the life energy your food is transferring to your body and ask your body to digest it with ease. This is magic for the way your body responds to food, try to do this every time you eat, in your own special way. Eating should be a ritual, providing your body with life energy is symbolic, tap into this spiritual aspect of feeding your BeUtiful body.

Before you sleep tonight, take a moment to quietly sit in your own space, peaceful and calm, no rush or hurry, close your eyes and gently begin to visualize your body bathed in light, notice what color the light is and feel it nourish and nurture you. See your body looking radiant and glorious, see what you look like when you are connected with U, how BeUtiful you are when you are aligned with who-you-really-are, enjoy this sense of wellbeing and enjoy feeding your mind positive energy.

Before you sleep, write whatever comes to mind, sleep early and rest.

Day 3 - Rest your Soul

Before you get out of bed this morning, lay on your back and close your eyes again as you connect with your breath. Breathing deeply and peacefully, listen to your body. Take your attention to your feet, then draw your attention up your body toward your ankles and then your knees. Take your attention further up toward your thighs, hips and your tummy, feel your breath in your tummy. Then move ever further up to your heart, feeling your heart open and your lungs breathing. Feel your neck, relaxing in the softness of your pillow and your head, clear and light. Take a moment to be aware of your body in this moment. Now, ask your body if there is anywhere that needs your attention? If something comes to mind then direct your attention there, you could even place your hands over that area if you can reach, and be mindful of this through the day. If nowhere came to mind then just relax and enjoy the moment.

As you open your eyes, what are you appreciative of in this moment? Keep this feeling of appreciation with you for the day.

For the final day of your ritual, give yourself a rest from the outside world, cleanse your mind as you cleanse your body. Take the emphasis away from watching TV, checking Facebook or Instagram and being so available on email or what's app. Instead, be with yourself.

Your focus for the day is to simply Be. Explore how aware you can be, in the moment, when you are preparing your food for example. Are U preparing your food, or are you on autopilot and your awareness elsewhere? Give even the simplest of tasks your undivided attention.

Drink your hot water as normal, sipping gently, feeling the hot water flow through your body. Light your favorite incense or a candle and sit comfortably in front of it, with your eyes half open rest your gaze on the flame. Watch how the flame moves, the color's that it glows, see how it dances. After a few moments, close your eyes and keep the image of the flame in your mind's eye. Keep watching to see what it does now, breathing deeply and completely. When you are ready, open your eyes and stretch your body.

As you go through today, consider what your experience has been over these three days, what has your experience meant for you, what feelings have been unearthed, what thoughts have been percolating, what inspirations have you had?

At the end of the day, take a moment to Be present and thank yourself, and your body, for going through these three days. Feel the peace that you have nurtured during this ritual, become more familiar with this sense of peace and know that you can connect to it at anytime.

Have an early night and rest.

The following morning, ease yourself into the day gently. Your digestive fires have loved the rest and the rekindling process has begun, so eat intuitively with extra care for the following few days. Drink plenty of water, eat simple food as you allow yourself time and space to transition.

Week 6 - Let GO

BeUtiful Mantra - I gracefully let go of everything that is weighing me down and I easily feel lighter.

Now your digestive fire is burning bright it's time to focus on letting go of all the heavy feeling accumulation, toxins and negativity that you no longer need, physical and emotional, cleansing these toxins by energizing your liver.

Remember, your liver metabolizes fat, therefore a strong liver is essential to allow your body to work through heaviness and toxicity so you can feel lighter.

If you are still enjoying the previous weeks then stay there until your body lets you know it's time to move forward. It will be different for everyone so trust your own instinct. When you are ready...

Cleanse your Mind - Let go of negative thoughts, especially about food and your body. This week become more conscious of the thoughts running through your mind. If you catch yourself thinking a negative or unloving thought then remind yourself that you have the ability to continue, or to choose another thought that is more loving. You are what you think. If you want to feel light, you must learn to think light thoughts!

Intuitive Eating - Really important this week as we introduce more foods that specifically support the liver and aid in letting go. There is a little transitioning involved here, building on the previous weeks, so you must do this at your pace, in your body's timing, not necessarily by the book!

Eat Liver Healing Foods - Coconut, cinnamon, turmeric, carrot juice, beetroot, artichokes, chicory, watercress, leafy greens, garlic, broccoli, cauliflower, cabbage, grapefruit, lemon, lime, avocado, walnuts, dandelion tea and milk thistle tincture. Incorporate these foods into your daily eating in a way that feels good for your body. Remember the Pendulum test, start using this if you feel you need extra help to guide your choices.

You don't have to do everything, just pick out the things that sound good for you and your body. It is tempting to want to do everything, but trust your body. A little goes a long way and a little of what's right for you does wonders. For example, having a carrot juice twice a week, taking a milk thistle supplement, and starting to cook with coconut oil (it is actually the most stable of the oils at high temperatures), this would be a great start. Just choose one liver loving thing to do each day, simple as that.

Your liver is associated with the emotion of anger. Become aware if you are holding on to any angry feeling energy, either directed toward yourself or someone, or something else. Each morning choose to do something that actively supports your liver, and remind yourself of your ability to let go.

This Week's Foodie Inspiration

(see www.lovebeu.com for all recipes)

Breakfast:

Golden Mylk Porridge

Mango & Turmeric Lassi

Be Cleansed Juice

Lunch:

Let Go & Let Goddess Salad

Be Light Soup

Smashed Avocado with Lime & Chili on Toast

Dinner:

Cauliflower Coconut Rice

Garlic, Kale & Artichoke Buckwheat Pasta

Love your Liver Stir Fry

Week 7 - BeU Ritual; Love & Light

BeUtiful Mantra - I connect with my heart and feel the love and light that I am.

Your spleen is nourished, your digestion is flowing, and your liver is totally loved up, especially after the Love your Liver Stir Fry! You're absorbing all the good stuff and letting go of all the other stuff, feeling lighter by the day.

Now you're going deeper, into your heart, with a three day BeUtiful Heart Ritual, blending body, mind, and soul as you transcend the physical and fine tune your alignment with your true self. There is beauty in Being U. Now I want you to feel it.

Traditionally, fasting allowed for higher connection to yourself and the universe, and was undertaken as part of a spiritual practice. This BeUtiful Heart Ritual will cleanse your body, mind and soul. The intention of this ritual is focused on bringing more love, light and healing energy into your heart, creating space for more love to be felt, both for yourself and others, whilst releasing heavy emotions of sadness and guilt. Remineralizing and rejuvenating, infusing your cells with high vibrational vital life force energy, seeing the light so you may feel the light.

Choose three days when you can be as free from other obligations and distraction as possible. Doing this type of cleansing ritual whilst you are busy and under pressure, can cause more harm than good, so gift yourself time, or wait until the time is right for you.

On the eve of your Ritual prepare yourself for the next three days, ready your mind and body for the change in your daily routine. Welcome the change and be excited about what these three days will gift you and your BeUtiful body.

Love & Light Ritual

(see www.lovebeu.com for all recipes)

On waking: Large mug of hot water with fresh lemon

Breakfast: Be Light Juice

Mid-Morning: Be Love Smoothie

Lunch: Be Easy Green Smoothie

Mid Afternoon: Ceremonial Hot Cacao

Dinner: All Loved Up Soup

Stay well hydrated, drinking up to 3 liters of room temperature, pure mineral water.

Where attention goes energy flows, whilst you are eating the foods above please follow this guidance.

Daily Love & Light Guidance:

As you awaken, remain still for a few moments and allow yourself to come gently into the day. Say good morning to yourself, and welcome you and your body into this wonderful day.

Start your day with your water and lemon, sit in your favorite spot and enjoy sipping this as you appreciate the goodness that it brings to your body. Once you have finished your tea, make yourself comfortable, in whatever position feels good and take a moment to pause.

Now open your heart, literally, raise your arms straight out in front of you with your palms facing together. As you take your next inhale, open your arms as wide as you can taking them as far behind you as is comfortable, on your exhale draw them back together as you bow your head to your heart. On your next inhale, open your heart again with your arms as wide as they can go and bring them softly together as you exhale and bow your head to your heart. Repeat this twelve times before you rest your arms and stay still to feel the wonderful effect of opening your heart.

Close your eyes and begin to deepen your breathing so you can hear it, listen to your breath, what story is your breath telling you today? Remain here for fifteen minutes if you can, practicing meditation and listening to the story of your breath.

Enjoy your juice and practice mindfulness as you drink slowly and calmly.

Walking in nature is such a powerful tonic for body, mind, and soul. It doesn't matter which part of the day you choose, just when it feels good for you is fine, but get outside and into nature. A beach, a forest, open fields, a beautiful park, even your garden, get out there and surround yourself with natures energy. Walk, gracefully, mindfully, consciously stepping one foot in front of the other, feel the ground beneath your feet as it supports your body, feel the air that wraps around your body, notice your surroundings, appreciate the naturalness of where you are and walk, slowly, gracefully and mindfully.

Before you sleep, open your BeUtiful Body journal and ask, what was in your heart today? Begin to write anything that comes to mind, let the energy from your heart flow as it pours onto the page in front of you. Do not judge, just allow it to flow.

As you go to bed, thank your body for doing such a wonderful job today, appreciate what you have been able to experience, being out in nature and enjoying the pleasure of being. Intend to rest well and sleep.

Repeat this for each of the three days, following the menu and this daily guidance, taking everything nice and easy, being gentle with yourself and most importantly cultivating a sense of mindfulness and deep connection with yourself.

On the eve of day three, take a moment to appreciate yourself for completing these three days and for having the courage to open your heart. Honor the journey you have taken to get to this point, and...

"Be realistic... plan for a miracle!"

Osho

Week 8 - Be Light

BeUtiful Mantra - I love myself unconditionally, I feel at peace within my skin, I am LIGHT. By now you will be feeling more balanced, lighter, and with a greater sense of ease in your body. Now you must build upon this because there is no turning back. Instead, focus on integrating what you have experienced so far with your new understanding, awareness and appreciation of your body and food.

For this week, and indeed, every week to come, I want you to stay connected with yourself, eat intuitively, be conscious of how your body is feeling and stay true to all that you have experienced and understood on this journey. It now becomes a daily practice of self-love for your BeUtiful Body, and realizing the true power of your thoughts and intentions to create.

Think LIGHT Thoughts - All healing begins in the mind. Now more than ever you have to focus your mind on light feeling, positive thoughts. This takes discipline, but now you are more conscious of yourself this will be much easier to practice daily. Make a choice to focus your mind on loving thoughts about yourself and your body, and commit to this daily.

Feel LIGHT - Each day practice love for your body, incorporating all the tools you have learned for this, on a daily basis. Practice appreciation for your body, strengthen your awareness of your body and connect with yourself each and every day. Love is a verb as well as a noun, action speaks louder than words, how are you loving your body today, and everyday?

Intuitive Eating - Go back over these past few weeks and take your foodie inspiration from these menus, mix and match depending on what feels good, before, during, and after eating. This is the perfect time to move deeper into your practice of intuitive eating. Becoming conscious of the subtle differences that occur depending on which foods you eat together, how much sleep you got last night and how stressed you're feeling today.

BeUtiful Body Basics - Keep it clean, keep it natural, drink plenty of water, don't skip a meal, eat slowly, chew properly, and listen to your body! Simplicity makes it easier to be consistent, and it's consistency that will make the difference.

What You Visualize You Materialize - Allow yourself the freedom to create, and keep your eyes focused on what you want. Feel your way through this, and in feeling it, know that you are! Imagine what it feels like to feel light, to feel beautiful, to feel comfortable in your skinny jeans, see yourself breathing deeply and with ease, at peace in your skin, owning the beautiful Being that you are right NOW by virtue of you being U. Use your imagination and embrace just how powerful you are!

Now is your time to shine, to enjoy the connection with your inner self and to eat and BeU! Eat intuitively so that your food is always working to create balance and harmony within your entire system. This will make you feel more grounded, more connected. Eat intuitively so you are free from bloating, free from heaviness, free from sugar rollercoasters, free from guilt and free from stress, so it is just U. This is the spirit of eating to BeU.

In the beginning, I said that beauty is in Being U. All we have done has been to facilitate an inward journey, clearing away the toxins and heaviness on all levels, and allowing your beauty to permeate through your subtle layers for you to create your most BeUtiful body.

Now you are clearer, and more connected to your own inner voice and body wisdom. This is what is going to propel you further, always expanding and never looking back on your old ways of dieting and body shaming, remember your BeUtiful Promise!

Anytime that your digestion feels lacking in fire, you know exactly what to do to get this going again. If you have a period of extreme stress and you feel completely ungrounded, you know what to do, go back and support your spleen. Don't be afraid to do this, act on your intuition, respond to your own biofeedback. Learn from your experience of these 8 weeks, what felt good, what worked, what didn't, hear the wisdom your body wants you to know.

Part 8 - Be LIGHT

It is time to Be the light that you are, and this section gives you practical tips and advice to help you with this every single day, and remember, this is a daily practice of mindfulness and unconditional self-love. It is a choice, moment by moment, to either stay with yourself and create peace, or leave yourself behind and create stress. There is beauty in simplicity and power in consistency. All of these tips are simple, which means you can be consistent with them and experience their power.

Sun LIGHT

The sun's energy is vital for life and our health. Some people have even mastered using the sun's energy as their sole source of nutrition, living on only water and sunlight – fascinating!

We need not go to that extreme but the truth is that the sun provides vital nourishment for the body, it stimulates the pituitary gland, energizes your cells, aids vital functions and can lift depression. For example, sunlight allows the synthesis of Vitamin D, which among other things, is essential for calcium and phosphorus absorption, healthy growth and development, immune function and reducing the likelihood of depression.

The sun provides 'light' energy that infuses into each cell, piercing through density and heaviness, bringing more 'light' into your body and allowing your vibration to rise, powerfully contributing to your vital life force energy.

Get outside, daily, fifteen to twenty minutes twice daily is optimal according to research. If you can, try to go sunscreen free, especially chemical sunscreens, as this just puts extra stress on your liver and loads your systems with unnecessary chemicals. Early morning and late afternoon, when the sun is not too strong is the best time to get your sunlight. If you can't do this then definitely consider a Vitamin D supplement, liquid D3 is the best I have found for absorption capacity.

Breathe Deep

The quality of your breath, that is, how well you breathe, directly informs your brain under which state to function, either one of peace or stress. If your breath is short, erratic and shallow then this tells your body to operate under a state of stress and your body shuts down non-essential systems, conserving energy for 'fight or flight' in response to the imminent threat or danger. Conversely, breathing deeply and calmly with full inhale and exhale, informs your brain to operate in a peaceful state and promotes openness, flow, proper digestion, and therefore, lightness, just as Dr. Bruce Lipton's research tells us. It is that simple, but incredibly profound, because it means you have control of your entire system literally within your breath.

"By changing patterns of breathing, we can change our emotional states and how we think and how we interact with the world."[29]

Therefore, breathing deeply is one of the most fundamental, basic, practices that you can do, right this moment, that yields infinite positive benefits for you and your body. And, if you want your body to feel light, breathing well is a necessity.

Mindful breathing also helps you to 'come back into your body', to feel grounded, balanced and centered. It oxygenates your system, which enhances vitality and helps everything to function as it should. Dull and dry skin can be the result of poor oxygenation in the body, as can nervousness and anxiety. Simple breathing techniques can provide the necessary environment for your body to heal these conditions.

Build 15 minutes of mindful breathing into your daily routine, you don't have to be sat with your eyes closed meditating to do this, you can mindfully breathe whilst showering, blow-drying your hair, driving or walking your dog. It doesn't matter when or how you do it, it just matters that you become conscious of the quality of your breath and make the conscious choice, daily, to breathe well and feed your body the energy it needs to self-heal, thrive and Be light.

Beauty Sleep

Beauty sleep, the importance of which we are tirelessly reminded of when we look like we could use it! It is a beauty basic and essential for feeling light in your body.

If you have been stressing about your body not 'behaving', and by that I mean not responding to your best exercise and eating efforts, or feeling more anxious or heavier than usual, then not enough sleep is a likely cause. In fact, to create your most BeUtiful Body, a good night sleep is an essential, not a luxury.

Sleep regulates your entire system. It allows for healing, restoration, balancing and cleansing. It also resets your body every day, free from the stresses and strains of the previous day to avoid accumulation, on all levels. Without enough sleep you will undoubtedly feel heavy, you will crave sugary foods, find your appetite challenging to address in a healthy way, your skin will not be as radiant as it naturally could be, you may feel more sensitive, anxious and irritated, it could even affect your hormones creating more challenging monthly cycles.

Sleep literally restores lightness and peace throughout your entire body whilst boosting your immune system and soothing your adrenal glands. There really is beauty to be found in sleep, so, if you are going through sleepless nights here are some of my favorite remedies and tips:

» *Avoid caffeine after lunch. Caffeine can actually have a prolonged effect on your body, meaning a mid-afternoon coffee which seems harmless enough can wreak havoc when it comes to bedtime. Keep all caffeine to the morning if possible.*

» *I love Rescue Remedies Night time drops. They are totally natural and I find them very relaxing. I know many clients who have had positive benefits from other Bach Flower remedies too so these are worth trying.*

» *Valerian Tea I find more helpful than Chamomile, in fact, Chamomile does not help me sleep at all. If it does for you then great, but if not try Valerian Tea or drops.*

» *Your evening meal should be warm, comforting and calming foods. Think root vegetables, soups, sautéed vegetables, lentil dal and stews. All of these foods do not over stimulate your system and their warm grounding element helps your body to relax. Avoid raw foods like salads, excessively spicy foods or rich foods at night.*

» *Minerals are essential for proper sleep, in fact issues sleeping could indicate a deficiency, specifically in calcium and magnesium. Both of these relax the body and promote better sleep. Try to include more mineral rich foods in your diet like dark leafy greens, pumpkin seeds, sesame seeds, avocado, banana, nuts, beans and lentils. Cacao is extremely rich in magnesium so a hot cacao drink is a tasty option!*

» *B vitamins are also vital, specifically B6 and B12 as they help to prevent insomnia. Try eating sunflower seeds, fresh fruits and vegetables, nutritional yeast, quinoa, oats, lentils and nuts. B12 supplementation is strongly recommended to obtain optimal levels.*

» *Tryptophan is an amino acid that helps to regulate and induce sleep and is essential for maintaining a proper sleep cycle. The highest plant based sources are buckwheat, mint leaves, nuts, seeds and legumes.*

» *Read in bed rather than watching TV or scrolling down FaceBook. Reading gets me every time but if I am watching TV or playing with my iPhone, sleeping feels impossible as my mind is so easily stimulated.*

» *It is important to create an environment conducive for rest and relaxation, where you can feel safe and protected, so make sure your bedroom has comforting elements like dim lights, cosy blankets and is a quiet place where you really do feel safe.*

» *If I really can't sleep I sit up in bed, legs out stretched, pillow resting on my thighs, then I forward fold and rest my forehead on my pillow. This is a yoga pose that is incredible for insomnia, and it works! Stack the pillows as high as you need them to be comfortable in your forward bend. Close your eyes, breathing fully and deeply, stay there for 5 minutes, then gently raise yourself up and lay down to sleep.*

» *Set an intention. The more you obsess about not sleeping the worse the problem is going to get. Your mind is incredibly powerful, it creates your internal environment and ultimately determines your experience. So guide your mind by setting a positive intention to sleep easy.*

Color Healing & Food

Nature is multi-colored and each color, according to science, has a differing effect on human mood and behavior. Colors have the ability to calm or energize, warm you up or cool you down, de-stress or invigorate, help you to sleep or wake up. They can even influence your appetite, as many food label designers know!

The power of color has long been acknowledged, as far back as the Ancient Egyptians, they used colors in their paintings to create different emotional effects on people. Colors are essentially energy, vibrating at different frequencies, hence their impact on us.

Interestingly in food, different colors indicate different vitamins, minerals, phytonutrients, and antioxidants. This is when 'eat a rainbow a day' comes into effect, as it's great way to make sure you're getting the full range of nutrients your body needs. Simply put, the more colors you eat the more diverse your nutrient intake is.

If you infuse color awareness into your intuitive eating then you can be confident that your diet contains a broad range of nutrients. It's a really simple, and easy, way of choosing what to eat and engages your senses allowing your body wisdom to communicate what it needs most and when. It maybe the red of the strawberries that gets your attention, or the bright green garden peas or rocket or the wonderful deep purple of a plum or blackberry.

Eating by color opens a channel of communication between you and your body that is easy to understand and based upon instinct. It's uncomplicated, empowering and accessible to most, including children. Look at the color of the food you eat in a day, is it multicolored or monotone?

Colors stimulate your chakras too. Chakra's are energy, colors are energy and food is energy, and it's all interacting in your body. Therefore, eating foods of certain colors stimulate the chakra with the corresponding color as its vibrational frequency resonates with that chakra.

For example, the heart chakra is connected to your heart organ and is usually associated with the color green. So, eating green foods is a great way to strengthen your heart chakra as the color resonates with that energy. Interestingly, green foods are typically full of the mineral magnesium, which happens to be one of the most important minerals for a strong and healthy heart. Ginger, when peeled, is a beautiful golden yellow color that corresponds with your Solar Plexus. This governs your digestive fire and ginger is excellent for making that fire stronger and stimulating digestion.

Notice the colors that you are drawn to, and allow this to be different day by day, meal by meal. Feed yourself with color.

Be The Light Ritual

Now you have gone through the 8 week experience of creating your BeUtiful body, whilst you are incorporating all lessons learned, I want you to assign one day per week to U! Not that every other day isn't all about U, but life gets busy and we live fast, so coming home to yourself one day each week acts as an anchor to keep you feeling balanced and connected.

Fasting is one of the most powerful healing tools, with each ancient medicinal model having some form of fasting practice. Apparently, there is nothing fasting can't heal if you fast for long enough! It sounds mystical, but modern science now supports what spiritual healing practices have been doing for thousands of years.

Intermittent fasting has received quite a lot of attention lately for being an excellent way to lose weight. However, if you just 'cut calories' on specific days, you are completely missing out on the real meaning and transformational power of this practice, which is an opportunity to quiet your mind, bring your senses inward, rest your body and allow a process of restoration, repair and rejuvenation to take place, physically, emotionally and spiritually.

Fasting essentially is a spiritual practice. Embrace it in its entirety and not only will you reap all of its rewards, it will be an easier, more comfortable experience, for you.

Choose a day that feels good and that fits with your schedule and lifestyle, remember to work with yourself rather than against, take the path of least resistance!

Here is an example of what to eat during your Be The Light ritual day. You will find options and recipes on my website so feel free to mix and match, and remember, keep listening to your body! Drink as much water as you comfortably can, warm water and teas like nettle and green tea, or whatever you feel drawn to.

Be The Light Ritual

(see www.lovebeu.com for all recipes)

On Waking: Water Ritual

Breakfast: Nourishing smoothie

Mid-Morning: Coconut Water or Vegetable Juice

Lunch: Green Smoothie

Mid Afternoon: Herbal Tea

Dinner: Mineral 'Frequencies of Light' Vegetable Broth

Stay well hydrated, drinking up to 3 liters of room temperature, pure mineral water.

On this day keep exercise to a minimum, walking or yoga is fine, but nothing too strenuous. Focus on flexibility and movement rather then full-on working out.

Meditation is key to fully embrace the benefits of this ritual. Take the opportunity to 'witness' yourself, practice your mindful breathing and sit quietly in meditation before breakfast for 15 minutes. Fasting is not just a physical process, it is a spiritual, mental and emotional one. If you know and appreciate what you are doing and why you're doing it, you will gain tremendous insight that will transform your life and your body! This day is really about creating space for you to connect more fully with All that you are and to Be inspired, so that you can integrate the wisdom gained into your everyday life and quite literally 'Be the light'.

Intuitive Exercise

A healthy body needs to move, as much as I've been talking about rest and relaxation, it's all about the balance between movement and stillness, and working intelligently with your body to find what that balance is for you.

Movement gets your juices flowing and stimulates digestive fire as well as your lymphatic system. A body that is always still easily becomes stagnant, and energy accumulates making you feel lethargic and heavy.

Flexibility is also important for a healthy, light feeling body. If your joints and muscles are stiff then energy is not able to flow freely. Regular stretching creates 'space' in your body and feels good because it helps your body let go of tension, both physical and emotional. Your 'issues' are in your tissues, so stretching these out is a great way to encourage feeling lighter. Yin yoga is amazing for this, and well worth a try if you feel inspired.

You are unique and will have a different combination of activities, and intensity levels, that will work for you. The most important factor is that you enjoy what you are doing. Just like eating, you need to feel good before, during, and after exercising. This way, you know that it is contributing to your wellbeing and helping you to feel lighter in a sustainable way.

If you are not loving your exercise regime then stop and take a moment, is there something else that would feel better? Staying fit and healthy is not about punishing your body in a grueling gym workout, quite the contrary, and this causes more harm than good. Also, you must be conscious of your monthly cycle and work-out with your hormones Alisa Vitti describes how to structure exercise for best results according to where you are in your cycle on her website[30], and I have found this incredibly useful. Specifically because I also suffered from adrenal fatigue and thyroid issues. Exercise can completely sabotage your best efforts at a light feeling body if it isn't done intelligently. Forget the 'no pain no gain' attitude if you also suspect adrenal fatigue, it will make you heavier! Slowly and gently is the way to go, but Alisa describes this wonderfully so check out her site.

If you dread exercise then your body is trying to tell you that there is a better way that is more suitable for you, and when you find this, you will get the results you are looking for. Not only that, you will be doing something you enjoy. Your enjoyment feeds your soul and spills out into other areas of your life. Before you know it, you are feeling good!

Exercise has been a tough lesson for me, and on many occasion I have been forced to rest because I'd ignored my body screaming "no more" at me for too long. I would just keep going, training like a woman possessed, but going nowhere fast. I ignored my body and dragged myself to the gym or out running, even when I would feel seriously tired or unwell. It's funny when I look back, but I never got the hint that I just needed more rest and perhaps another form of exercise, I made it such hard work because I believed it had to be!

I am not saying that exercising is bad, or working up a sweat and getting out of breath is something you should avoid. Not at all. If it makes you feel good before, during and after then great, keep it up. But I didn't, I dreaded it before I got there, dragged myself through it and then felt more exhausted after.

I urge you to be conscious of how your body feels about exercise, and be confident in the knowledge that you will get the results that you desire quicker and easier, if you do what feels good. You will be more consistent and this is the key, a daily practice of working with your body.

When done in the right way for your body, exercise will boost your serotonin levels, improve your mood, raise your confidence, make you feel strong and empowered. Intuitive exercise is powerful as your body actually begins to respond to the exercise you do, getting stronger and lighter, rather than weaker and heavier!

Reconnect To U

I remember when I first had the experience of consciously feeling connected with my body. I was in a yoga class with time to spare before it started, and I was just sitting waiting, stretching a little. As I had my head resting on my knees, I started to consciously breathe, like you do in a typical yoga class. Then, in that moment, my hands were gently touching my legs and it occurred to me that I had never really paid attention to my body before.

How crazy, I thought to myself, because most of my time was occupied thinking about food, exercise, my body, weight, shape, and size. In my head, I thought my body had my upmost attention since I thought of nothing else. But in those few quiet moments, I realized that I had never actually connected with my body properly before this moment.

I had been in my head, not in my body. Everything had been going on in my mind, it had nothing to do with my actual body, or reality for that matter. For the first time, I saw that all that I'd been telling myself was more to do with my fears, poor self-esteem and my own disconnection from me, than it was reality. For the first time in those quiet moments, I was in tune with my body and I could feel it, something I had never felt before. This experience has made it so much easier for me to ignore all the chatter in my mind about not being good enough, not looking good enough, feeling heavy and un-attractive.

Get out of your head and feel your body, feel your own touch, feel the sensation of your attention on your body in a loving way. Feel how wonderful and comforting that feels, and how a warmth of emotion rushes over you as you find that space - that quiet time to connect to your body and the wholeness that you are.

You are worthy, you are deserving. Listen carefully to your body wisdom, trust it, trust yourself and honor your journey. Connect with your inner self, be still, nourish your divine feminine nature, find your balance and enjoy your most BeUtiful body.

Now You're Awake

If you've been reading between the lines, you will realize what is really at stake here. It goes far beyond your body. This is your life.

Don't let yourself be distracted by anything that doesn't have your wellbeing at heart. Ask yourself, do the gossip magazines body shaming well known females have anyone's wellbeing at heart? Does the latest diet fad consider your wellbeing when they make guarantees about their product being the answer to all your diet nightmares, selling caffeine fuelled diet pills or food products full of everything but real food? Or a food and drug industry hell-bent on their bottom line at the expense of your health and wellbeing?

Nothing is at it seems and the more you are influenced by marketing campaigns and what's trending on social media, the more you get distracted. From what? From U, and this is the problem that we face today.

The BeU philosophy, and everything we have been talking about in this book, is a movement focused on helping each of us to reconnect with ourselves, reclaiming our sovereignty and personal power to challenge the status quo that right now needs to be challenged, not just for women, but for all human beings and our wellbeing.

Whilst you're busy not loving your body, not loving yourself, not feeling good enough and not trusting your own intuition and body wisdom, your health and wellbeing suffers. All of your amazing potential stays trapped inside and God knows we need your amazingness to be out here, all singing and all dancing, being the change that you seek.

The sooner we wake up to our true beauty, the sooner we will be able to transform not just our inner world and physical body, but our outer world and the life that we are living. This is my vision for us all.

"As above, so below, as within, so without."

Alyson Noel

To BeU is BeUtiful.

With LOVE.

Resources

Balch, P. A. (2006). Prescription for Nutritional Healing Fourth Edition. London: Penguin Group.

Bruyere, R. L. (1989). Wheels of Light. California: Bon Productions.

Carroll, L. J. (2005). The Architecture of Abundance. London: Piatkus Books Ltd.

Chopra, D. (2001). Perfect Health. London: Transworld Publishers.

Cousens, G. (2005). Spiritual Nutrition. Berkeley: North Atlantic Books.

Eden, D. (1999). Energy Medicine. London: Piatkus Books Ltd.

Emoto, M. (2007). The Healing Power of Water. Hay House.

Grotto, D. (2008). 101 Foods That Could Save Your Life. New York: Bantam Dell.

Hanh, T. N. (2006). Understanding Our Mind. California: Parallax Press.

Hauck, D. W. (1998) Food Alchemy. Retrieved June 4 2011 from http://www.alchemylab.com

Hay, L. L. (2004). You Can Heal Your Life. Hay House.

Hicks, J. a. (2008). The Amazing Power of Deliberate Intent. Hay House.

Holford, P. (2004). New Optimum Nutrition Bible. London: Piatkus Books Ltd.

Hurley, L. (n.d.). Foods that Weaken the Spleen. Retrieved September 1, 2009, from Alternative Health: http://www.alternative-health.ie

Jensen, B. (1983). The Chemistry of Man. Escondido: Bernard Jensen International.

Leaf, C. (2007). Who Switched Off My Brain. Dallas: Switch on Your Brain.

Legget, D. (n.d.). Food Energetics The Spleen. Retrieved August 16, 2009, from Meridian Press: http://www.meridianpress.net/spleen.html

Marley, J. (n.d.). Liver in Chinese Medicine. Retrieved August 16, 2009, from Acupuncture Services: http://www.acupuncture-services.com

Mateljan, G. (n.d.). Retrieved December 20, 2009, from The Worlds Healthiest Foods Web site: http://www.whfoods.com/

Stossier, H., & Frith Powell, H. (2009). The Viva Mayr Diet. London: Harper Collins Publishers

(Endnotes)

1. Statistics on Weight Discrimination, A Waste of Talent, The Council on Size and Weight Discrimination, www.cswd.org

2. Adrian F. Heini, Divergent Trends in Obesity and Fat Intake Patterns: The American Paradox, The American Journal of Medicine, 2007

3. Three out of Four American Women Have Disordered Eating, Survey Suggests, Science News, www.sciencedaily.com (2008)

4. Weight Loss and Weight Management Market Forecast to 2019, www.marketsandmarkets.com

5. Childhood Obesity, US Department of Health and Human Services

6. National Association of Eating Disorders

7. Statistics on weight Discrimination: A Wastes of Talent, The Council on Size and Weight Discrimination

8. Davison & McCabe, 200; Birbeck, 2003; Stice et al, 2000; Phares et al, 2004

9   The Human Body In Symbolism - http://www.sacred-texts.
        com/eso/sta/sta17.htm

10   Trans Fats: The Science and the Risks. WebMD.

11   The Good Gut: Taking Control of Your Weight, Your Mood
        and Your Long-Term Health, by Justin Sonnenburg and Erica
        Sonnenburg, PhDs.

12   Defining the Human Microbiome, by Luke K Ursell, Jessica L
        Metcalf, Laura Wegener Parfrey, and Rob Knigh

13   Vagal   Pathways   for   Microbiome-Brain-Gut   Axis
        Communication, by Forsythe P, Bienenstock J & Kunze WA.

14   The Good Gut: Taking Control of Your Weight, Your Mood
        and Your Long-Term Health, by Justin Sonnenburg and Erica
        Sonnenburg, PhDs.

15   www.nutritiontotheedge.com - The Blood Sugar Rollercoaster

16   www.nutritiontotheedge.com - The Blood Sugar Rollercoaster

17   Dr. Axe - www.draxe.com

18   Heather Hausenblas, Ph.D., Associate Professor of Exercise
        Psychology, University of Florida, Gainesville

19   Judith Wurtman, Ph.D., former director of the Research
        Program in Women's Health, Massachusetts Institute of
        Technology Clinical Research Center

20   Rate of Eating Disorders in Kids Keeps Rising, US Department
        of Health and Human Services

21   The Stress and Cancer Link: 'Master-Switch' Stress Gene Enables
        Cancer Spread, Ohio State University, Professor Tsonwin Hai

22   www.medicalnewstoday.com - Oxytocin: What is it and what does it do? MNT

23   Dr. Jonas Frisen, Karolinska Institute in Stockholm, Cell 2005 Jul15;122(1):133-43

24   www.meridianpress.net - Introducing the Spleen, Daverick Leggett

25   Nature experience reduces rumination and subgenual prefrontal cortex activation, published in Proceedings of the National Academy of Sciences

26   Ascension Glossary

27   wikipedia.org

28   www.medicinehunter.com - Holy Basil: Relieve Anxiety and Stress Naturally

29   Yoga Breathing, Meditation, and Longevity by Brown RP and Gerbarg PL, 2009

30   www.floliving.com - Alissa Vitti